How to Lower High Blood Pressure

How to Lower
High Blood Pressure

The Natural Way to Reduce Hypertension

Dr Caroline M. Shreeve MB,BS (Lond)

Thorsons

Thorsons
An Imprint of HarperCollins*Publishers*
77–85 Fulham Palace Road,
Hammersmith, London W6 8JB

The Thorsons website is: www.thorsons.com

Published by Thorsons as
Lower Your Blood Pressure in 4 Easy Stages 1989
High Blood Pressure 1993
This edition revised and updated 2001

10 9 8 7 6 5 4 3

A catalogue record for this book
is available from the British Library

ISBN 0 00 712094 X

Printed and bound in Great Britain by
Creative Print and Design (Wales), Ebbw Vale

Contents

Introduction

Yes you *can* reduce your blood pressure naturally and safely! Proven self-help methods can often reduce a mildly or moderately raised blood pressure unaided, or enable your doctor to prescribe lower doses of drugs should these remain necessary.

Claims to cure 'blood pressure' overnight have been made in the past by catch-penny charlatans whose miracle remedies turn out to be a disappointing waste of money. You will find no claims for miracle cures in this book. The information it contains is based upon the results of scientific studies and upon the established usefulness of a number of complementary (i.e. alternative) therapies.

If you are in your 20s or 30s and have — so far as you know — perfectly normal blood pressure, you may think of hypertension (abnormally raised blood pressure) as a complaint of older people. Certainly the average blood pressure in Western countries does rise with age; but far from being normal, this is a reflection of our lifestyle and a major risk factor in the development of heart and arterial disease.

Recent research has shown that the blood pressure readings of some overweight children and teenagers equal those of many middle-aged adults. Hypertension produces few if any symptoms in its early stages, so take the precaution of having your blood pressure checked every six months. Follow the lifestyle hints in this book to keep your blood pressure within acceptable limits, and improve your vitality and well-being.

If you are already a sufferer, the combination of a healthier lifestyle and natural remedies will help to relieve your disorder and increase your chances of a fuller, longer and more enjoyable life.

Part one

Diagnosing
High Blood Pressure

Chapter one

Problems with Medication

'I'D RATHER AVOID DRUGS, DOCTOR...'

Do you suffer from high blood pressure? If not, then this book will help to reduce the chances of your doing so in the future. If you don't know, have your blood pressure (BP) measured and use the 'Four Easy Stages' to keep your BP within healthy limits. And if you are a sufferer, then you will probably identify with one of the following scenarios:

1. you take blood pressure medication as prescribed and go for regular BP checks
2. you take the prescribed tablets when you remember; you're not convinced that you need them and you rarely have your blood pressure checked
3. you've stopped taking the tablets because you feel just as well (if not better) without them.

Why All this Fuss?

It can be extremely difficult to convince someone who feels perfectly fit that they need to take medication for the rest of their lives. This is particularly true when their raised BP was first spotted 'accidentally' during, say, a routine health check or insurance medical. Most GPs are fully stretched dealing with the common minor ailments of daily practice, as well as acutely ill patients and others with ongoing conditions such as emphysema or diabetes. So why do we worry about patients in groups (ii) and (iii) whom we rarely see from one year's end to the next?

The reason is that high blood pressure (hypertension) is often a silent killer, preparing the way without warning to kidney failure, heart attacks and strokes. Deaths from cardiovascular (heart and blood vessel) disease in developed countries rise annually, increasing numbers of men and women below the age of 40 are affected, and the percentage of women sufferers has risen since 1970. Growing numbers of families are affected by the invalidity or death of a dad or mum caused by high blood pressure which, for whatever reason, has remained untreated.

What about Side-effects?

The definitions of normal and high blood pressure, how high your blood pressure can be allowed to rise before you need treatment, and the rationale underlying the choice of drugs are covered in Chapters 3 and 4. Essentially, a blood pressure reading that may cause concern in one person may be normal – or at any rate acceptable – in another; age, gender and general health all have to be considered. Here we will look at the side-effects blood pressure medication can cause, and at practical problems relating to its use.

'Water Pills' (Diuretics)

These drugs are generally safe, and at least one from the many available is likely to suit you. They continue to work after the increased urine production (diuresis) subsides, and enhance the effects of other blood pressure medications prescribed with them. Most of them, however, cause loss of potassium in the urine, which can make you tired, weak and drowsy or, where the loss is severe, an abnormal heart rhythm (arrhythmia) can result. This is especially likely to affect elderly people who frequently eat insufficient potassium-rich foods such as meat, milk and milk products, and fresh vegetables and fruit, especially tomatoes and bananas.

Diuretics can also cause nausea, vomiting and diarrhoea (which, if prolonged, in turn will aggravate the potassium loss), as well as faintness, pins and needles, cramps and itchy rashes. Men taking them may have difficulty in sustaining an erection. Many increase the blood fat (cholesterol) level, a major factor in the development of clogged arteries (*see Atherosclerosis, Chapter 3*), and affect uric acid metabolism, increasing the risk of gout. Being seriously overweight predisposes you to a high blood sugar and diabetes, and these may be aggravated by diuretics, which is yet another incentive for you to shed surplus pounds. Examples of diuretics linked to potassium loss include Aprinox, Diurexan, Hygroton, Navidrex, Nephril and Lasix, also known by its generic name of frusemide and prescribed in many hospitals because it acts quickly and effectively when a large fluid loss is urgently required, and its effects can readily be monitored; and the thiazide group, such as bendrofluazide (Aprinox, Berkozide, Inderetic, Neo-naclex).

Potassium-sparing diuretics overcome the problem of mineral deficiency by reducing the amount of potassium removed by the kidneys. They can, however, cause most of the other side-effects associated with this class of drug. Potassium-sparers can be used on their own, but are often combined with other diuretics in compound medications. Examples are amiloride (Amil-Co, Burinex A, Fru Co, Frumil, Kalten, Lasoride,

Moducren, Moduret-25, Moduretic, Navispare) and triamterene (Dyazide, Dytide, Kalspare, Triam-Co). They can be the diuretic of choice for patients with liver failure or on digitalis heart drugs (e.g. Digoxin, Lanoxin), in whom potassium deficiency might cause serious complications.

Beta Blockers

Some people taking 'beta blocker' drugs also get tummy upsets and skin rashes, a slow pulse, cold hands and feet, and sleep disturbed by vivid dreams. Cold hands are a particular problem in elderly people, who are less able to cope with the drowsiness, confusion and poor sleep that can result.

Like diuretics, beta blockers can worsen blood sugar control in some diabetics on insulin or drugs such as glibenclamide (Malix, Calabren, Euglucon) or chloropropamide (Diabinese). They reduce the 'helpful', high-density variety of cholesterol known to help combat arterial disease, and can cause air tube spasm. They have to be prescribed with caution for wheezy or asthmatic patients and, for more complex reasons, for people suffering from heart failure.

Some people on beta blocker drugs may experience dryness of the eyes, although this was much more likely to happen with practolol, which is no longer available. This makes the eyes itchy and uncomfortable, and is a major nuisance if you wear contact lenses. Examples of long-established beta blockers − also known as 'first generation' − include propranolol (Beta-Prograne, Inderal, Inderetic, Inderex) and oxpranolol (Slow-Trasicor, Trasicor and Trasidrex).

Second-generation beta blockers such as atenolol (Beta-Adalat, Tenormin), bisoprolol (Emcor, Monocor) and metoprolol (Betaloc, Lopresor) work more selectively upon the heart, and have less of an adverse effect upon blood fats. Third-generation beta blockers e.g. celiprolol (Celectol) and nebivolol (Nebilet) which act on the peripheral circulation, have no such adverse effects on cholesterol. The case for beta blockers gets increasingly complicated as new members are added to this popular anti-hypertensive group: more about how they work and why they are chosen for certain patients in Chapter 4.

Vasodilators

Examples of vasodilators are hydralazine (Apresoline); minoxidil (Loniten); and diazoxide (Eudemine).

Hydralazine causes a rapid heart beat (*tachycardia*), flushes and headaches. Doses above 100mg daily can produce a condition resembling the auto-immune disease systemic lupus erythematosis or SLE, in biologically susceptible people (mainly Caucasian women). The symptoms include skin rashes, fever and painful joints and muscles.

Minoxidil causes rapid heart beat and tissue swelling (*oedema*) due to salt and water retention. It cannot be used to treat hypertension due to *phaeochromocytoma* (*see Glandular causes of hypertension, Chapter 2*), and its promotion of hair growth on the face, body limbs and elsewhere makes it unsuitable for women. It is now also marketed as Regaine, a clear yellow liquid applied to the scalp to treat pattern baldness (*alopecia androgenetica*), in men only.

Diazoxide can cause nausea, high blood sugar, tremors and abnormal muscular movement. All these drugs can precipitate *angina* in patients with coronary heart disease (*see Chapter 3*).

Calcium Antagonists

You will find all you need to know about the working of this widely prescribed and effective group in Chapter 4. I will just briefly say here that three Classes now exist, and that verapamil (Cordilox, Univer) in Class 1 can precipitate heart failure in people who also take beta blockers or suffer from certain types of electrical conduction defects of the heart.

Class 2 members, e.g. amlodipine (Istin), nicardipine (Cardene) and nifedipine (Adalat, Beta-adalat, Coracten, Tensipine-MR) do not depress the heart's electrical conduction or contractility, and are therefore less likely to trigger cardiac failure, although headache, palpitations, flushing of the skin and swollen ankles (due to their action on peripheral blood vessels) can be troublesome. The Class 3 calcium antagonist diltiazem (Adizem, Dilzem XL, Slozem, Tildiem and Zemtard XL) can slightly slow the heart, and cause flushing and dizziness.

ACE Inhibitors

ACE stands for 'angiotensin converting enzyme' (*see pages 24–25*). Examples are captopril (Capoten), enalapril (Innovace) and the recently introduced, once-daily lisinopril (Carace, Zestril).

They have fewer side-effects than many other antihypertensive drugs; those that do occur can include a sudden, dramatic fall in blood pressure (hypotension), a persistent dry cough, rashes, headaches, fatigue, dizziness, nausea and vomiting. Loss of taste (which returns to normal when the treatment stops) and angioneurotic oedema (swelling of areas of skin, mucous membranes and underlying tissue) have both been reported, but ACE inhibitors are generally well tolerated by the patients for whom they are prescribed.

Captopril can cause pruritis (itching), rashes, a cough and mouth ulcers. Enalopril can produce muscle cramps, urticaria (nettle rash), tiredness and nausea; and lisinopril may cause lethargy, weakness and chest pain.

ACE inhibitors can cause taste disturbances which may be counterproductive in people already off their food; and the first dose can seriously lower blood pressure in anyone on diuretics or suffering from dehydration. They also have to be prescribed with caution for patients with renal artery stenosis (depleted arterial blood supply to one or both kidneys), or with other forms of renal malfunction; and they are usually considered unsuitable for use during pregnancy.

ANGIOTENSIN II ANTAGONISTS

These act slightly differently from the ACE inhibitors and do not cause the dry cough or swollen rash for which that group is known. Examples include candesartan (Amias), losartan (Cozaar, Cozaar-Comp) and valsartan (Diovan). They are a generally safe and useful drug group although side-effects can include backache and upper respiratory infections (Amias); gastric upsets and dizziness (Cozaar, Cozaar-Comp); and fatigue and mildly disturbed renal and liver function.

LESS COMMON DRUGS

The drug or drugs you are taking or want to find out about may not fall within the groups just described, so here are brief notes on the other available types. The first four have been available for years and are far less often prescribed than they once were; the final two are relative newcomers.

CNS Depressants

These include: alpha-methyldopa (Aldomet, Dopamet, Medomet); clonidine (Dixarit, Catapres); and reserpine (Serpasil). The first of these was used to treat elderly hypertensive patients in a trial carried out in 1985 by Professor A. Amery and his colleagues at the University of Birmingham, and favourable results were reported in The Lancet. Despite this, neither it nor others in the group are often used as starting treatment for high blood pressure, but alpha-methyldopa may be used to control severe hypertension or prescribed for a patient who has been taking it for years before the consultation. Side-effects can include depression, a dry mouth and stuffy nose, drowsiness and lethargy. Men taking these drugs occasionally experience erection problems. There have also been several reports of an increased incidence of breast cancer in middle-aged women treated with reserpine.

Adrenergic Neurone Blocking Drugs

Examples include guanethidine (Ismelin, Ganda), debrisoquine (Declinax) and bethanidine (Esbatal, Bendogen). They were among the first antihypertensive drugs to be taken by mouth, and made a very significant contribution to hypertension therapy in the 1950s.

The side-effects limiting their use include postural hypotension (sudden fall in blood pressure on standing up, often accompanied by dizziness); failure of ejaculation; nasal stuffiness; diarrhoea and constipation.

Ganglion Blockers

Ganglion blockers, e.g. trimetaphan (Arfonad), are used to treat hypertension associated with aortic aneurysm (an abnormal bulge in the side of the wall of the aorta) and are administered by intravenous injection (i.e. into a vein). Ganglion blocker side-effects include severe postural hypotension and the rapid development of tolerance (i.e. the need to give larger doses to achieve the same effect). They are usually only used during surgical procedures.

Chemoreceptor Depressant Drugs

Veratrum (Thiaver, Veriloid, Rauwiloid + Veriloid), the sole member of this group still available in the UK, is rarely prescribed because it tends to send the blood pressure plunging down and also to cause a high incidence of unacceptable side-effects.

Alpha Blockers

Examples include prazosin (Hypovase) and indoramin (Baratol). The initial dose of prazosin may be followed by severely lowered blood pressure. Indoramin has a sedative effect and can also cause severe postural hypotensive problems. Both can cause headaches and nasal stuffiness.

Alpha-beta Blockers

Labetolol (Labrocol; Trandate) is the first drug of this class to be marketed in the UK. Large doses can cause orthostatic hypotension.

PRACTICAL PROBLEMS

Whether you experience side-effects from your drugs or not, it is essential to remember to take them regularly. This can be a problem if you travel frequently, have a busy daily routine or simply have a poor memory. Opening screwtop bottles and tablet jars can be trying if you have arthritis in your hands. Container manufacturers, in their attempts to make their products childproof, seem to have forgotten that adults needing to open them may lack sufficient strength and dexterity. Even blister packs (the type in which the tablet or capsule is pushed through the metal foil backing of a card covered with clear protective wrapping) need a certain nimbleness of the fingers.

If you are elderly it is often very hard to remember to take tablets when prescribed. You may find that you have a bewildering assortment of medicines and pills of all shapes, colours and sizes, and find that you cannot read the small printed names and instructions on the container labels. Trying to think back to what the doctor said, while you wrestle unsuccessfully with a resistant bottle top, can cause a lot of anxiety.

Some senior citizens living alone make out lists (which it is easy to get wrong!) and set their alarm clocks to remind them that it is 'pill time' – the days seem to revolve around the next dose. If you cannot remember what the doctor said each kind was supposed to do for you, it is often tempting to forget about them and leave them to collect dust.

A better idea is to get your doctor to explain again and again, until you are certain you know exactly what you have been prescribed, and why. If your eyesight is reasonably good, then ask the doctor or the practice nurse to write the instructions down in clear handwriting or print.

The 'placebo' effect some medications can have, despite a mistaken view of what they have been prescribed for, was illustrated by tablets I once prescribed for an 80-year-old man. He thanked me profusely when he had finished the three-week course, saying that the stomach upsets, poor appetite, heartburn and hiccups which had bothered him for years had disappeared entirely. Puzzled, I consulted his notes, and found that when he had seen me earlier, he had complained of swelling and pain in his arthritic knee joints, and that in fact he had been taking the non-steroidal anti-inflammatory arthritic drug Feldene (piroxicam)!

Potassium supplements often cause confusion. These may be prescribed with certain water pills to replace reduced stores of this mineral (*see above*). If an elderly or confused person cannot relate them to any of his or her symptoms, then the point of taking them is not apparent.

Potassium supplements are sometimes added to the water pills themselves, removing the need for extra pill-taking. Others are supplied as a whole tablet, or as granules which make up a sparkling drink when mixed with water. However palatably they are presented, though, they often cause gut irritation and nausea.

If you suffer from bladder problems, getting to the toilet in time can be a nightmare when you are taking diuretic drugs. Public toilets seem to vanish from the earth's surface when you are out shopping and need to visit one urgently. If you are elderly or handicapped and house-bound, it can be just as difficult. Negotiating furniture and maybe long corridors in a hurry, when your walking difficulties make you frightened of falling, may result in your passing some urine before you reach your destination. This is extremely distressing, causes a lot of extra washing and ironing, and is one of the major problems of water pill treatment for anyone with limited mobility.

Among the practical difficulties you may face from the side-effects of blood pressure drugs are lethargy and drowsiness. These can affect your work, especially if you have a sedentary job in a warm, close atmosphere; or they can cause you to sleep during the daytime if you are house-bound, thus disturbing your night sleeping pattern.

Nausea, stomach pains and diarrhoea can make you feel weak and debilitated, as well as putting you off your food; and giddy spells are especially dangerous if you drive, handle dangerous machinery, or are elderly or handicapped and alone. Headaches, stuffy nose, cold hands and feet, erectile problems, skin rash, poor sleep and eye dryness can also make you miserable.

The advice that follows should help to relieve both the side-effects and the practical problems of blood pressure drugs, if you have to continue taking them in addition to the self-help methods described in this book. Reassure yourself at this point that, even if this is the case, your general health and fitness level will improve if you combine them with your medication. Indeed, you may well find that you can reduce your blood pressure satisfactorily without having to rely on prescription medicines of any kind.

Swallowing Medicines

No discussion of the problems you can encounter with medication is complete without mentioning one of the commonest of them all – that of actually taking them. Many people find it difficult to swallow tablets of any type. This is most likely to be the case if you are elderly, suffer from a mouth or throat disorder, or have the type of gullet that seems to 'close up' the moment it meets a tablet or spoonful of medicine. In your experience, a spoonful of sugar is no help at all in making the medicine go down!

This problem can be partly psychological in some people, who have no problem at all in gulping half-chewed food, including hard, pill-sized pieces of salted nuts, boiled sweets or popcorn! Swallowing tablets and capsules is also difficult if you feel sick (as a result of the last dose?!), are recovering from an illness, or have a poor appetite. Dainty morsels may well slip down the 'red lane' with comparative ease, while medication leaves you gagging. Save one such treat as a reward for taking after medication, and drink plenty of water.

PROGRESS REPORT

You now know something of the wide variety of side-effects and practical difficulties high blood pressure sufferers may encounter with standard drug treatment. It is only fair to say that some patients experience no adverse reactions at all; and it is extremely unlikely that anyone would be affected by all the 'nasties' a particular drug is capable of causing.

If you are being treated for hypertension, you *must* remain on your course of tablets until the natural techniques you will learn about here produce a measurable improvement. It is then that your doctor will consider reducing the dose, or taking you off your tablets for a trial period. If you do experience adverse reactions to any drug, the right thing to do is to return to your GP and ask for a change of prescription to something that suits you better. Even if you have to stop taking medicines because they do not 'agree' with you, you need a substitute.

We should also acknowledge the hard work pharmaceutical scientists and doctors, over the past four decades, have put into testing new formulae and carrying out clinical trials with a view to improving the effectiveness and acceptability of antihypertensive drug treatment. It is fashionable to criticize the pharmaceutical industries harshly for the millions of pounds they earn yearly, but consider where we would be without adequately researched medication and innovatory pharmacological products.

The drugs containing rauwolfia alkaloids, obtained from the south-east Asian shrub *Rauwolfia serpentina*, are a case in point. They were among the earliest of the antihypertensives to be used. Originally prescribed as sedatives, they were found to lower raised blood pressure, and the first to be prepared, reserpine (Serpasil and Serpasil Esidrex), has been used in this capacity for decades. The other rauwolfia drug is methoserpidine (Decaserpyl, Decaserpyl Plus).

These drugs act on the hormone adrenaline contained in nerves. They are prescribed far less often nowadays, which is just as well because they can cause a stuffy nose, tiredness and diarrhoea, as well as an increased production of stomach acid (to be avoided at all costs if you have a peptic ulcer).

Another unpleasant reaction to both rauwolfia and the vasodilator drugs is postural hypotension, which makes you feel giddy and unbalanced for a few seconds on suddenly standing up, perhaps even leading to a fall. Severe depression, which in some people leads to suicidal tendencies, has also been reported in patients taking rauwolfia.

It is interesting to contrast the situation when rauwolfia compounds were the mainstay of antihypertensive treatment with the greatly improved medical facilities doctors now have at their disposal. In 1986, a report appeared in a doctors' weekly newspaper bearing the headline, 'Life expectancy boost for blood pressure victims.' It stated that medicine had scored a 'remarkable victory over malignant hypertension' (a very serious condition, *see Chapters 3 and 4*) 'with the possibility of near-normal life expectancy'.

The report reminded readers that 25 years earlier, the five-year survival rate in patients with retinopathy (damage to the retina of the eye due to an abnormally high blood pressure often causing blindness, and indicative of life-threatening hypertension) was less than 1 per cent. Professor John Swales and his colleagues at the Leicester hypertension clinic were now reporting five-year survival figures of 82 per cent of the first 100 patients with very serious retinopathy seen at the clinic since it began in 1974. This figure approaches the five-year survival rate for the general population of 94 per cent.

Perhaps an even more impressive outcome was mentioned in the same newspaper article, of a group of Spanish kidney specialists (diseased kidneys are a major cause of malignant hypertension) who had studied 165 affected patients between 1974 and 1984, and reported an 87 per cent five-year survival. The reduced death rate among the patients with damaged kidneys depended to a considerable extent on the early treatment of kidney failure. All the same, a great deal of success at both centres was due to the use of drugs to control the dangerously high blood pressure, 'most patients requiring three or more drugs in combination to do so'.

The advantages of the wide range of differently acting antihypertensives, which attack the problem from a variety of angles, are clearly underlined by this report.

The same newspaper carries an interesting feature on the 'striking success' in the management of high blood pressure achieved by an open-access clinic at Stobhill General Hospital using a number of innovations. These included adequate consultation time, flexible appointments, nurses to carry out routine tests, and individual advice to patients about diet and giving up smoking.

Of the 500 patients attending the clinic, 175 had been attending for four years. Good blood pressure control had risen from 22 per cent to 79 per cent. The results were achieved primarily on a simple regimen of a beta blocker in 70 per cent of the cases, combined with a diuretic if necessary. Only one third of the patients needed a vasodilator drug as well.

Disappointingly, though (the writer added), the clinic approach had not influenced either smoking habits or weight reduction in severely overweight patients.

My point in including the last piece of information is not to imply that smoking and being overweight are not seriously harmful, particularly for hypertension sufferers, but to point out how much better even these admirable results might have been, had the patients complied with the advice they were given. Many of them would very probably have been able to keep their own blood pressure within healthy limits without the help of drugs, or at least to have their doctors reduce their medication doses. The goals of treatment and when it should be started differ in some respects in the UK from guidelines issued in the United States and by WHO (World Health Organisation) (*see Chapter 2, page 30*).

Vital messages cannot be repeated too often; and I will say again here that *all* cases of hypertension must be diagnosed and dealt with. Before describing the many things you can do to reduce your own blood pressure (as well as precisely how to go about them!), it is necessary to explain what blood pressure actually *is*, why it is essential to life, and how, when seriously raised, it can cause grave organ damage and death.

Chapter two

What *is* Blood Pressure?

You must have heard people say, 'I've got blood pressure'. It is a very good job that they have, since without it they would be dead! A critically ill or injured patient rushed into hospital has his or her blood pressure checked immediately by the casualty officer or nurse, and a low or absent (i.e. unrecordable) reading indicates a state of severe shock. Restoring it to normal is a vital, life-saving procedure.

People really mean that they have a *raised* blood pressure, which can be equally life-threatening in the long term. Its potential for harm can best be understood through acquaintance with the normal circulatory pressure, the factors that regulate it, and how it can get out of control.

HOW THE BLOOD CIRCULATES

Our 5 litres (about a gallon) of blood are driven around the body by the heart, a two-sided pump. Blood drains into its right side from the veins and is directed to the lungs, where it gives off carbon dioxide and picks up a fresh supply of oxygen. It then enters the left side of the heart, and is recirculated around the body. En route, waste material is removed by the kidneys, and digested nutrients are picked up from the stomach and small bowel.

Blood flows from the heart to the periphery of the body in arteries. The largest of all is the *aorta*, which comes off your heart just behind the top of your breast bone, giving off big supply branches to your neck and arms. It then runs down inside your chest and abdomen in front of your backbone, giving off further branches, and finally divides in your pelvis into the right and left femoral arteries that supply blood to your legs.

This system is like a road map, with the aorta as the motorway, giving off 'A-road' arteries to important towns. You can easily locate these by feeling your pulse at various points. The large brachial artery in your arm produces a 'thrust' on the inside of your elbow joint.

The carotid arteries running up your throat can be found pounding away an inch or so on either side of your Adam's apple. If you get frightened or excited and your heart starts to race, you usually become aware of their throb. Unless you are very fat, their pulse can be seen below the surface of your skin, and helps to give the game away about how you are reacting!

If you feel deep within your groin with your finger tips (don't dig too hard!), you will feel your femoral artery, the source of supply to your thigh and calf muscles, your feet and toes.

All these 'A-road' arteries give off smaller 'B-roads' to the various organs and muscles between which they pass. They, in turn, divide into even smaller ones, ending up as little unclassified roadways, the arterioles, which finally divide into the tiniest of all the vessels, the capillaries. These form a vast network of minute footpaths and bridle tracks with a diameter of about 1/100 millimetre (0.01mm) and run through the tissues themselves.

Blood delivered to the capillaries by the arterioles is rich in oxygen and essential nutrients (e.g. glucose, amino acids). These pass out through the capillary walls into the surrounding tissue fluid and so to the cells. Under normal conditions, large protein molecules and blood cells remain within, although the white cells are capable of getting through when they need to. When injury or invading bacteria cause inflammation, histamine is secreted by the damaged cells and the walls of the capillaries leak. Extra fluid from the plasma, white cells and occasionally red cells then escapes into the surrounding tissue spaces.

As oxygen and nutrients pass out of the capillaries, carbon dioxide and other waste products of cellular metabolism pass in. The capillaries link up with small veins (venules) which join to form larger and larger vessels on the way back to the heart and lungs. In this way, capillaries are both the end of the arterial system and the start of the venous (vein) system, and form a vital bridge between the two.

The discovery of the capillaries was made by Marcello Malpighi, 17th-century professor of medicine and anatomy at Bologna and Pisa, and the first professional anatomist to work with a microscope. Malpighi's breakthrough was a highly important extension of William Harvey's discovery of the circulation of the blood in 1628. Harvey realized that blood travelled continuously around the body but, having to base his observation and deductions entirely upon what he could observe with the naked eye, he could not identify the means by which blood passed from the arteries to the veins.

Harvey's findings marked the end of the era of ancient medicine and the beginning of modern medical science. Malpighi's contribution set the scene for a vast increase in our understanding of anatomy, physiology and cellular metabolism.

The Nature of Blood Pressure

In a healthy person, the pressure of the blood leaving the heart is around 120 mm of mercury, i.e. 2.4 lb per square inch. Because the motorway and A-road arteries are wide, the flow of blood within them meets little resistance, and its pressure is largely unaltered. The arm artery is chosen for measuring its value, both for this reason and because it is easily accessible to the doctor's blood pressure cuff and stethoscope.

The B-road branches are narrower, but there are enough of them to prevent a 'traffic hold-up' of blood in the A-roads that give rise to them.

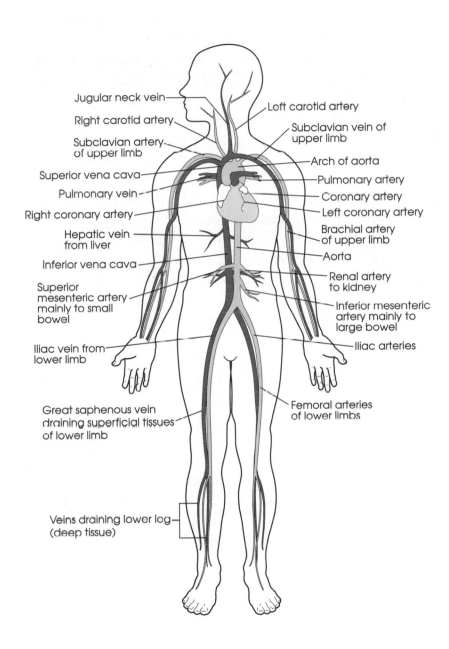

Jugular neck vein

Right carotid artery

Subclavian artery
of upper limb

Superior vena cava

Pulmonary vein

Right coronary artery

Hepatic vein
from liver

Inferior vena cava

Superior
mesenteric artery
mainly to small
bowel

Iliac vein from
lower limb

Great saphenous vein
draining superficial tissues
of lower limb

Veins draining lower leg
(deep tissue)

Left carotid artery

Subclavian vein of
upper limb

Arch of aorta

Pulmonary artery

Coronary artery

Left coronary artery

Brachial artery
of upper limb

Aorta

Renal artery
to kidney

Inferior mesenteric
artery mainly to
large bowel

Iliac arteries

Femoral arteries
of lower limbs

However, the pressure of the blood falls progressively as the routes get more and more narrow, and the arterioles offer the greatest resistance to its flow. By the time it reaches the capillaries, it measures only about 32 mm mercury. Because the capillaries are so minute, they might be expected to offer the greatest resistance of all; but there are so many of them that they offer less than the arterioles. The drop in pressure across the capillary network is only around 20 mm mercury.

The pressure in the veins is practically nil, i.e. it is about equal to atmospheric pressure. Blood from the lower half of the body would be unable to overcome the pull of gravity and reach the heart if it were not for a number of special help factors.

One of these is the massaging effect of surrounding muscles – especially important in the veins of the legs, whose valves play an important part in preventing backflow. Another is the increase in negative pressure that develops within the chest cavity as we inhale and encourages the flow of blood along the veins in the direction of the heart.

Why We Need Blood Pressure

The function of blood pressure is to maintain a flow of blood to every part of the body, most importantly the brain. Unlike other organs, its needs never vary, and they remain at around 750 ml of freshly oxygenated blood per minute, regardless of whether we are sleeping or waking, working or relaxing.

Temporary interference with the brain's supply, e.g. when blood pools in the legs during a long period of standing still, causes a fainting attack. Consciousness is soon regained as the person falls to the ground or places the head between the knees, since either action restores the brain's blood and oxygen supply.

A cardiac arrest, however, is a state of the greatest emergency requiring immediate resuscitative measures. When the heart ceases to beat, the circulation of the blood comes to an abrupt halt and the blood pressure falls to zero. Irreversible brain cell damage and death occur if oxygen is lacking for only three minutes.

While abnormally low blood pressure causes uncomfortable symptoms and can be fatal when extreme, significantly raised blood pressure strains the heart and blood vessels, can cause serious damage to other organs, and greatly increases the risk of heart attack, strokes and other disorders. It is therefore very important to identify high blood pressure (hypertension) in its early stages, and prevent it from rising to a dangerous level.

HOW BLOOD PRESSURE IS MEASURED

The heart pumps the blood in spurts. With each beat, it squeezes or contracts – the phase called 'systole', pronounced *sys-tol-ee* – to eject its blood into the arterial system. This pressure, around 120 mm Hg (mercury) in a normal person, is known as the systolic pressure. The heart then relaxes – 'diastole' (*dye-as-tol-ee*) – and fills up with a fresh supply of blood.

The blood pressure is prevented from falling to zero, and the flow of blood is prevented from reaching a standstill between beats, by the elastic composition of the arteries. Their walls are stretched every time the heart beats (systole), pumping blood into them, and they rebound as it relaxes during diastole. This ensures a steady stream of blood around the circulatory system at every phase of the heart's action, and keeps the pressure during diastole at around 80 mm mercury.

The sensation of force which you feel when you take your pulse is due to the difference between systolic and diastolic pressure, and is normally around 40 mm mercury.

The blood pressure is measured by means of a sphygmomanometer, the original version of which was invented by the Italian physician Riva-Rocci in 1896. There are many sophisticated modern forms but they are all based upon the principle deduced by the original designer. Its essential components are a column of mercury in a vertical, graduated tube marked in millimetres, balanced by the air inside an inflatable arm band or cuff.

This is wrapped around the upper part of the arm above the elbow. The head of the stethoscope is placed on the brachial artery on the front of the elbow joint, with the arm fully extended. The cuff is pumped up, and the point at which the sound of the arterial pulse disappears i.e. is suppressed by the (equal) pressure inside the surrounding cuff, is the systolic pressure.

The pressure in the cuff is then gradually reduced, and the lower of the two numbers – the diastolic BP – is the reading taken as the sound of the heartbeat via the stethoscope reappears.

HOW BLOOD PRESSURE IS CONTROLLED

Besides the elastic recoil of the arteries, two other factors regulate the blood pressure, namely the rate at which the blood flows, and the resistance to that flow offered by the blood and its vessels.

(1) The *flow* of the circulating blood is adapted by complex nervous and chemical means to meet prevailing demands. After a meal, the autonomic nervous system – responsible for the automatic, unconscious control of bodily functions – dilates the arteries supplying the stomach and small intestine. This brings extra blood to that area to cope with the digestive processes, and is compensated by the narrowing of arteries elsewhere in the body whose demand for blood is less immediate.

When we are threatened, frightened or angry, the stress hormone adrenaline, released by reflex action from the adrenal glands, makes the heart beat faster and diverts the blood from the skin and other areas to the limb muscles. This explains the white-faced look typical of anger or terror, and prepares us for the primitive danger reaction of flight or fight.

The flow also varies enormously according to a person's state of activity. It is usually around 5 litres a minute at rest, and may be five or six times this amount during prolonged aerobic exercise such as cross-country running when the heart is beating very rapidly.

(2) The ability of the blood flow to change so readily, in response to the body's minute-by-minute needs, emphasizes the importance of *resistance* to the flow in maintaining a stable blood pressure. The thickness (viscosity) of the blood is partly responsible, i.e. the thicker a liquid, the harder it is to pump along a narrow channel. Normally, the blood's thickness does not change, which means it is the calibre of the blood vessels themselves that is largely responsible for blood pressure regulation.

This brings us to the arterioles, which are all-important in determining whether the blood pressure remains safely within the range of normality, or whether it zooms skyward, threatening health and life. We have seen the significant part the arterioles play in lowering the pressure of the blood as it passes through them to the capillary network. Their diameters vary according to whether their muscular walls are relaxed or constricted. This is determined by impulses arising in a group of nerve cells – the vasomotor centre – located in the lowest part of the brain, and reaching their muscular walls via the autonomic nervous system.

If the heart's output of blood decreases (e.g. after a sudden haemorrhage), the consequent fall in blood pressure is counteracted, at least in part, by constriction of the arteriolar walls. When the blood flow from the heart increases, it is necessary for them to relax slightly, in order to keep the blood pressure steady.

If for any reason they fail to do so, then either the flow within them must be reduced or the pressure inside them must rise. The heart continues to maintain a steady flow of blood to meet the body's requirements, however much resistance it meets. Consequently, if the calibre of the arterioles is too narrow, it simply pumps harder to overcome the obstruction. The flow continues as normal, at the cost of the blood pressure, which consequently rises.

The kidneys also play a part in blood pressure control. They are highly dependent upon a constant supply of blood, and when this is reduced, they react by releasing an enzyme, renin. This is converted in the blood into the chemical substance angiotensin, which causes the walls of the arterioles to contract, thereby raising the blood pressure and restoring the kidneys' supply of blood.

DEFINING HYPERTENSION

High blood pressure is so common, and can have such serious consequences, that the term 'hypertension' might be expected to have a precise meaning. In fact, health experts have expended a great deal of effort in their search for an acceptable definition.

A wide range of blood pressure values has been obtained from human population studies. When these values are plotted as a graph, there is invariably a skew towards higher ones, but no natural or obvious break separates normality from abnormality (*see Fig. 2*). For this reason, the definition of hypertension remains empirical, i.e. it can only be arrived at through constant observation and experiment.

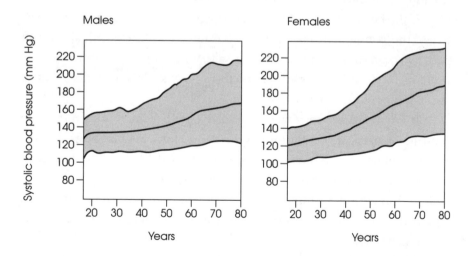

Like normal body weight, normal blood pressure has come to be recognized as that which is statistically associated with the greatest life expectancy. It is the level at which the heart and circulatory system are best able to carry out their work, and at which the risk of developing heart disease and other related disorders are lowest.

The systolic blood pressure may rise by as much as 50 per cent in healthy people when the blood flow increases in response to extreme emotional excitement or very vigorous exercise. It quickly returns to its resting level, however, and the diastolic pressure remains more or less unaltered throughout. The latter is the more important of the two. It reflects the condition of the arterioles, and an abnormally high reading means that they are constricted, their narrower than normal interior channels offering increased resistance to the flow of blood within them.

People with blood pressure of 170/110 mm mercury and above frequently experience symptoms such as morning headaches, fatigue and dizzy spells; and those with values above 230/130 mm mercury are highly likely to develop heart failure or other serious conditions. The greatest risk to anyone with a significantly raised blood pressure is the sudden and apparently unpredictable catastrophe of a heart attack or a stroke.

Hypertension is not a disease in the usual sense of the word, but it is the most important criterion by which doctors can predict the likelihood of future heart or circulatory disorders. It is also a risk factor that can be controlled both by antihypertensive drugs and by self-help methods.

THE CAUSES

Specific causes of hypertension can be found in only 5–10 per cent of patients. This means that they are all relatively rare but details are included here for the sake of any blood pressure sufferers who may have had one of them diagnosed.

(1) *Chronic renal disease* causes the blood pressure to rise. It damages the blood vessels of the kidneys and reduces their blood flow. This results in the release of the hormone renin (*see above*) and constriction of the arteries. Conversely, diseased kidneys, e.g. from stenosis (narrowing) of the renal arteries, also causes hypertension.

(2) *Glandular causes* include thyrotoxicosis (overactivity of the thyroid gland); and malfunction of the outer shell of the adrenals, which produces excessive quantities of certain hormones affecting the blood pressure.

A very rare adrenal gland tumour – *phaeochromocytoma* – secretes large quantities of the stress hormones adrenaline and noradrenaline into the bloodstream, producing sudden attacks of very high blood pressure.

(3) *Narrowing* (coarctation) of a section of the aorta shortly after it leaves the heart (*see above*) produces high blood pressure in the head and arms, and low pressure in the rest of the body. Present at birth, this condition is commoner in males and generally produces symptoms such as headaches, nosebleeds and aching legs between the ages of 15 and 30. The only treatment is an operation to remove the narrowed section of the artery.

(4) *Toxaemia of pregnancy* is a cause of hypertension in expectant mothers. A slight blood pressure rise during pregnancy is common, but antenatal check-ups always include measuring the blood pressure, in order to make sure that it does not exceed 140/90 mm mercury. Should this occur, the patient's progress is carefully monitored for early signs of toxaemia. These include fluid retention, first seen as severe ankle swelling and excessive weight gain; and protein in the urine. Specimens are tested routinely throughout pregnancy for signs of this, and also for glucose, blood or other abnormal constituents.

If signs of toxaemia appear, the patient is watched carefully, and advised to restrict her salt intake, and to rest and remain as quiet as possible. Hospital admission is essential if the condition worsens, because *eclampsia* – a form of epilepsy – can occur at an advanced stage of pregnancy and threaten the life of both mother and child.

Women who suffer from toxaemia of pregnancy stand an increased risk of developing hypertension later in life.

(5) *An excessive number of red blood cells* increases the viscosity (thickness) of the blood, and thereby the resistance to its flow and the pressure of the blood. The normal number of red cells is around five million per ml (millilitre) of blood, and a figure above six million is considered abnormal and termed *polycythaemia*.

Loss of plasma from the blood such as occurs in burn injuries increases the red blood count, because although the actual number of red cells is unaltered, the volume of plasma in which they are suspended is reduced. Red cells *do* rise in number in response to oxygen shortage; this happens to people living at very high altitudes where the atmosphere is rarefied, and in others who suffer from severe heart and lung disease which prevents sufficient oxygen reaching the tissues.

In a rare condition known as *polycythaemia rubra vera*, the number of red cells can rise to nine or ten million for no accountable reason. Either some have to be drawn off, or the development of new red cells has to be prevented by means of drugs or radiation.

(6) *Certain drugs* can cause or worsen hypertension, including the contraceptive pill, steroids and non-steroidal anti-inflammatory drugs – NSAIDs – used to treat arthritis. The NSAIDs can cause fluid retention and a consequent rise in blood pressure.

Hypertension for which no cause can be found is called *essential* – a mild to moderately raised blood pressure is often symptomless, and only discovered by chance during a routine health check or insurance examination. A mildly raised blood pressure is not necessarily harmful in itself, but it can become more serious, and represent a serious threat to life expectancy.

Screening for Hypertension

Clinically significant hypertension carries the same degree of risk as a raised blood fat (cholesterol) level, and experts in hypertension management recommend screening to detect asymptomatic patients.

About two-thirds of adults consult their doctor at least once a year, and over 90 per cent are seen at least once every five years. Routine blood pressure measurements, carried out at consultation if no recording has been made during the past five years, are now recommended in men and women aged 30 to 70 years.

There is no need to postpone having your blood pressure measured, though, until you next have something wrong with you! Often it is unnecessary to see the doctor: practice nurses carry out many routine blood pressure checks nowadays, and the earlier a high value is detected, the better, particularly if you are aged 45 or over.

A systolic blood pressure above 160 mm mercury, or a diastolic pressure above 95 mm mercury, increases the risk of developing coronary heart disease by a factor of five, compared with someone of the same age and sex but with normal blood pressure.

A report of the third working party of the British Hypertension Society, 'Guidelines for the management of hypertension', was published in September 1999 by the Cardiovascular Research Institute, University of Leicester, Leicester Royal Infirmary. Here are its suggestions for the management of high blood pressure in people both with, and without, diabetes; all BP measurements are in millimetres of mercury.

1. *Lifestyle changes* should be implemented in *all* patients with established and borderline hypertension.
2. *Non-diabetics:* treatment should be started where there is a sustained systolic blood pressure of 140–159 or sustained diastolic between 90–99 in patients with a significantly increased 10 year risk of coronary heart disease, or with signs of existing damage to 'end organs' (the parts of the body that suffer most from the effects of

prolonged hypertension – the heart and blood vessels, eyes, kidneys). Treatment is also needed for patients with sustained rises of 160 or more systolic, or 100 or more diastolic.

3. *Optimum treatment target for non-diabetics* is below 140 systolic and a diastolic pressure below 85.

4. *Minimum acceptable control in non-diabetics* is below 150 systolic over 90 or less, diastolic.

5. *Diabetic patients with hypertension:* treatment should be started if systolic BP is sustained at or above 140, or diastolic at or above 90.

6. *Diabetic hypertensives:* optimal BP targets are under 140 systolic and under 80 diastolic.

7. *Diabetic hypertensives:* minimum acceptable level of control is below 140 systolic and below 90 diastolic.

Treatment: the currently favoured first-line approach to treatment is a low dose thiazide diuretic (e.g. bendrofluazide, Aprinox) together with a beta blocker e.g. timolol (Blocadren), atenolol (in Beta-Adalat). *In older people:* a diuretic and/or a long-acting dihydropyridine calcium antagonist (e.g. nicardipine – Cardene SR) are preferable to a beta blocker because of the many adverse effects the latter can have, such as narrowing of the airways (bronchospasm) and interference with the electrical current conduction of the heart.

Other drugs may also be prescribed to reduce high risk factors threatening the heart and blood vessels:

a. aspirin helps to keep the blood liquid and to guard against coronary thrombosis (heart attack) and stroke;

b. statin drugs such as cerivastatin (Lipobay), pravastatin (Lipostat) which reduce the total amount of cholesterol in the blood, usually prescribed for a cholesterol in excess of 5.0 (millimols per Litre); and

c. glycaemic agents such as metformin (Glucophage), to help control blood sugar levels in diabetics

RISK FACTORS

Blood pressure values fluctuate constantly. Stress is probably the commonest cause, and it is well-known that worrying that your blood pressure may be raised – a form of anxiety known as 'white coat syndrome' that reaches a crescendo as the pshygmomanometer cuff is wrapped around your arm – can rocket a normal blood pressure into the hypertensive range for the few important minutes involved in its measurement.

Few doctors prescribe antihypertensive drugs until a patient's blood pressure has been tested on three or four separate occasions. Patients who have rushed to the surgery for fear of being late are often asked to rest for 20 minutes to allow their blood pressure to subside. Orthodox blood pressure treatment is generally regarded as lifelong, and doctors prefer to be very certain that medication is necessary before starting therapy.

One theory about essential hypertension is that it results, in the early stages, from overstimulation of the sympathetic nerves (part of the autonomic nervous system) by prolonged exposure to stress and other factors. The resultant arteriolar wall spasm eventually causes structural changes that prevent these vessels from dilating in the normal way.

Certain factors, detailed below, are known to increase greatly the risk of essential hypertension developing.

Age

Blood pressure tends to rise as we grow older, the rate varying at different phases of our lifespan. There is a normal and fairly rapid increase from the low values of infancy to the higher values of childhood, adolescence and early adulthood, and graphs of the population's *average* blood pressure show a gradual, upward trend between the ages of 20 and 45 in both men and women, followed by a more rapid rise of 0.5 to 1.0 mm Hg systolic pressure per year until the age of 70.

It is possible, however, that the *normal* blood pressure increase between the early 20s and old age may be considerably less than is suggested by these findings. The majority of people develop some type of blood vessel disorder as a result of their diet, lifestyle or vulnerability to other risk factors, a fact to which their rising blood pressure gives testimony. The minority of people whose blood vessels remain disease-free throughout life show little sign of a rise in blood pressure as they age.

To claim that a person's blood pressure can be expected to rise from the age of 20 onwards is to claim that he or she can be expected to develop some degree of circulatory disorder or other kind of disease. Fortunately, even our risk-ridden, Western life style has not yet equated any type of illness – even those commonly affecting the majority of people – with normality.

Sex

Before you panic, this does not refer to sexual activity, but to gender! Hypertension in men is always more serious than in women, since their overall risk of developing heart or circulatory disease is greater. Referring to population averages, women have slightly lower blood pressure than men during their 20s and 30s, and slightly higher thereafter.

Possible reasons for this include hormonal changes, pregnancy, the use of steroid drugs such as the contraceptive pill and HRT (hormone replacement therapy) for menopausal symptoms, and perhaps a greater susceptibility to certain risk factors, such as weight increase, smoking, stress and alcohol intake.

Race and Environment

We are primarily concerned here with blood pressure problems in Western society. However, although most populations show an average

age increase and distribution of pressure values similar to our own, certain racial variations provide an interesting comparison.

Most population studies carried out in East and West Africa, the USA and the West Indies show similar proportions of hypertensive sufferers among black and white people, but some of the study samples indicate a considerably higher percentage among blacks. This contrasts with the results of studies carried out on the Indian subcontinent, where the number of hypertensive people is relatively low.

In some communities, the average blood pressure shows minimal tendency to rise with age – and the increase in blood pressure that does occur lacks the 'upward skew' of higher values found in Caucasians (*see Fig 2, page 26*). Examples include East African nomads, South West African bushmen, and certain Pacific islanders such as the inhabitants of Pukapuka in the Northern Cook Islands. It is possible that diet, exercise and an absence of the type of stress found in more developed societies provide a large part of the answer.

Obesity

Many studies have shown that putting on weight is associated with a significant rise in systolic and diastolic blood pressure, especially in young and middle-aged adults. Part of the reason is that, like every other body tissue, fat requires an adequate blood supply, and every pound of surplus fat increases the total length of the small blood vessels by approximately one mile! The heart is highly adaptable to many bodily changes, but the extra demands made upon it by a stone or more of excess fat are considerable.

Fortunately, loss of excess weight can reduce both high blood pressure in people suffering from hypertension and the chances of it developing in overweight people with a normal blood pressure. We will be looking at the safest and most reliable methods of weight reduction in Chapter 5.

Diabetes

The link between diabetes and cardiovascular disease is widely acknowledged. Diabetics run a greatly increased risk of damage to the heart and blood vessels, and for this reason are more likely to (1) develop hypertension, and (2) develop circulatory problems in response to raised BP. Diabetes doubles the risk of suffering from a raised BP. Hypertensive diabetics have an increased chance of disease to both large and small blood vessels and damage to the retina of the eye and the kidneys. If you have diabetes, make sure you are treated in accordance with requirements mentioned in the British Hypertension Society's Treatment guidelines, and that you attend frequent BP checks like clockwork.

Salt Intake

The relationship between salt (sodium) intake and hypertension is now well documented. Moderate and severe hypertension tends to improve on a salt-restricted diet, while reports upon the effects of this measure on mild hypertension are inconclusive. The safest approach, therefore, is to reduce our salt intake. You can either stop adding salt to your food; or you could use a potassium-rich substitute.

Chapter three

Hypertension and Health Problems

Hypertension is unusual, in that it is not an 'illness' in the usual sense, but a condition predisposing to the development of several disorders, some life-threatening. In addition, its early stages produce no symptoms; it rarely has an obvious cause; it can be controlled but seldom cured; it requires lifetime management; and the treatment itself may add symptoms.

One of the reasons that some doctors refrain from treating patients with mildly raised blood pressure is their reluctance to produce symptoms (i.e. drug side-effects) where none previously existed! Since all high blood pressure needs careful observation and control, the argument in favour of natural blood pressure reduction is particularly cogent.

It is essential to understand the risks hypertension imposes if you are going to make lifestyle changes to maintain or reduce its level. The younger you are, the greater the significance of a small blood pressure rise. If you are 35 and have a diastolic blood pressure of 100 mm Hg, your life expectancy is potentially reduced by $16^{1}/_{2}$ years. If you are 55, this same blood pressure predicts 'only' a six-year reduction in life expectancy.

Some doctors prescribe medication for hypertensive patients of all ages. Others treat only those below 65, because of the problems inherent in the use of certain drugs (*see Chapter 1*) and because some research studies suggest that elderly patients are unlikely to gain any real benefit.

Fortunately, natural methods to reduce and control blood pressure can be used by people of all ages. A reduction in life expectancy of six years for someone aged 65 *may* seem small to medical statisticians, but it can seem very great when you reach that age and hope to enjoy years of healthy, active retirement.

HYPERTENSION AND ILL-HEALTH

The disorders connected with hypertension are of two types. The first are largely the consequence of longstanding, abnormally high pressure inside the arteries, and include heart failure, kidney failure and strokes. The second are caused by the arterial disease atherosclerosis, the development of which is greatly accelerated by high blood pressure; they comprise coronary heart disease and peripheral vascular disorders.

Coronary heart disease refers to the ill-effects upon the heart of diseased coronary arteries. Peripheral vascular disorders affect the 'peripheral' blood vessels some distance from the heart, such as the femoral arteries and their A- and B-road subdivisions supplying the lower limbs.

Heart Failure

A moderately to severely raised blood pressure greatly increases the workload of the left side of the heart, which endeavours to pump as much blood as usual into the aorta and the rest of the arterial system against the increased resistance offered by the constricted arterioles.

Muscles – including those of the heart – grow bulkier when used to excess, and one of the earliest signs of heart strain is a thickening of the wall of the left ventricle, the lower, left-sided pumping compartment from which the aorta arises. Enlargement of the heart can be detected by a physical examination, by a chest X-ray and by an ECG (electrocardio-gram), an electrical tracing of the heart providing information about its size and performance.

Eventually the effort proves too much, and the left side of the heart shows signs of failure. The blood supply to the organs and tissues is decreased, causing weakness and lethargy. The build-up of pressure in the left ventricle prevents the blood from the lung veins from flowing freely into its upper compartment (atrium), which drains into it, rather like a heavy traffic flow getting held up in its passage from one main road to another already overburdened by rush-hour motorists. The lung tissue becomes congested, producing a cough and breathlessness.

The cough can be dry or produce frothy, blood-stained phlegm – especially at night when attacks of acute choking and gasping get patients out of bed and leaning out of the window, terrified that they cannot breathe. The breathlessness is first noticed during prolonged exercise. Later, it accompanies mild activity and, when heart failure is severe, patients become breathless at rest.

Unless the raised blood pressure is reduced, and the left-sided heart failure relieved, the right side of the heart becomes affected. Pressure builds up in the right atrium, creating back pressure in the veins draining into it. A characteristic sign of this is enlargement of the external jugular veins on either side of the neck, returning blood to the heart from the scalp and face.

Their superficial position below the skin of the throat, where they offer such a convenient target for vampire attack in horror films, also makes them especially vulnerable to injury. They are partly visible in healthy people en route to the heart, starting just below the angle of the jaw, crossing large neck muscles, passing on either side of the Adam's apple (larynx) and finally disappearing into the chest behind the collar bone. Swollen jugular veins congested by backflow pressure show characteristic signs which help doctors assess the severity of heart failure.

Other signs of right-sided heart failure, all consequences of a con-gested blood flow, include swollen feet and ankles, an enlarged liver, loss of appetite, a swollen tummy and passing less urine than usual.

Kidney Failure

The relationship between kidney disease and high blood pressure is a classic vicious circle. Kidney disorders, especially those which interfere with their blood supply, can cause hypertension. Conversely, persistently high blood pressure (particularly the malignant type: *see Chapter 4*) can injure the kidneys. It damages their arterioles and impairs their function, which is highly dependent upon an adequate blood supply.

Large amounts of protein are found in the urine in hypertensive kidney failure. Symptoms may include getting up at night to pass urine, and passing larger than usual volumes during the day. In kidney failure, toxic substances usually filtered off and excreted in the urine collect in the bloodstream. The patient's condition can deteriorate rapidly and death can soon result. Unfortunately, treating the underlying hypertension rarely improves kidney function.

Strokes

A stroke consists of damage to an area of brain tissue as a result of pressure from escaped blood or interference with the circulation and a consequent shortage of oxygen and glucose. Brain cells depend for survival upon a constant and adequate supply of these two factors, neither of which they are able to store, and significant depletion severely injures the affected area.

Hypertension increases the risk of a stroke in two ways. First it encourages the development of *atherosclerosis* (*see below*), thereby narrowing the arteries of the brain. This heightens their chances of becoming blocked by a blood clot from the heart or lungs, or by a flake of tissue arising in the heart or a diseased artery.

Secondly, it places severe strain upon the walls of the brain's delicate blood vessels, and can eventually rupture one of them. If it does, blood escapes into the surrounding tissues, constituting a cerebral haemorrhage.

Symptoms of minor strokes include loss of use of a hand, arm or leg and/or loss of speech. A more or less complete recovery is usually made within a fortnight, but lowering the blood pressure is mandatory.

Symptoms of major strokes can include weakness or paralysis down one or both sides of the body, speech loss and sometimes loss of consciousness. The brain damage, speech problems and paralysis persist for longer in a major stroke, but with help many people make a satisfactory recovery. Again, treating hypertension is a major priority.

Transient ischaemic attacks are similar to minor strokes and produce body tingles and numbness, speech difficulties, loss of awareness of identity and surroundings, lightheadedness and visual disturbances. They can be very frightening, but the symptoms are over within a few minutes. They are thought to result from temporary spasm of the blood vessels supplying an area of brain, or from pressure upon an artery in the neck carrying the brain's blood supply, as a result of getting the neck into an unsuitable position.

One third of people who experience a transient ischaemic attack have no further trouble; a third continue to experience them from time to time without suffering severe consequences; and a third eventually have a more serious stroke.

Senile dementia is the fourth leading cause of death in Britain, and it affects between 5 and 7 per cent of the population over the age of 65 and 20 per cent of those aged 80 and over. It impairs physical movement and thought processes, memory, energy, emotional stability, appetite and the ability and will to perform simple tasks such as dressing, preparing food or drink and reading or knitting.

There are several different varieties of this disease, the one most pertinent to a discussion of hypertension being *multi-infarct dementia*. A series of minor strokes, which escapes the notice of the patient and his or her relatives and doctor, gradually destroys areas of brain tissue. Hypertension strongly predisposes elderly people to this condition, and argues in favour of reducing raised blood pressure within this age group.

Atherosclerosis

The development of fatty lumps, or plaques, in the walls of arteries impedes the passage of blood within. This process largely accounts for the vast problems of coronary heart and peripheral vascular disease, and its course and causes have been researched intensively ever since its connection with heart disease became apparent.

Despite this, understanding of the highly complex process of atherosclerosis is as yet incomplete. It is not a single condition, but follows different sequences in different arteries. Fatty streaks appear in the lining of blood vessels soon after birth. During the first ten years of life, the lining thickens, and the small cushions of fatty material develop at points where the arteries branch.

These soft, yellow lumps reach maximal size and number between the ages of 20 and 30. One theory holds that they develop from a collection of monocytes – a type of white blood cell – which infiltrate the arterial lining, then engulf fat particles and other cells in their vicinity.

This sets the scene for the appearance of fibrous plaques, the hub of the atherosclerotic problem. Plaques start to appear in the arteries of susceptible people after the age of 20 and multiply as time passes, especially in high risk areas such as the coronary arteries and the cerebral arteries in the brain. They develop in the main from fatty streaks, a process which is sparked off, many experts believe, by some sort of damage to the arterial lining.

Blood flow turbulence is thought to cause this injury. Blood is pumped through the arteries at a rate of $1^1/4$ gallons (5 litres) every minute, under considerable pressure. Some damage – especially in key areas such as arterial junctions where turbulence is high – seems to be inevitable. High blood pressure appears to be the most important factor aggravating the initial damage to the delicate vessel lining.

Platelets – small particles present in blood – clump together on the fatty streak or another damaged area, with the object of repairing it. They release chemicals which turn a protein in the blood, fibrinogen, into solid, hair-like threads of fibrin. These carry the repair task a step further by entangling white and red blood cells within their meshes, like fish in a net.

The result is a clot. Under normal conditions this process is counter-acted, when it has gone far enough, by a powerful substance called *prosta-cyclin* produced by the arteries. This can be seen as a defence mechanism with which the arteries are equipped to prevent the formation within them of a dangerously large clot or thrombus. Sometimes, however, the platelets' repair facility becomes excessive. It overpowers the action of the prostacyclin, and a large thrombus is formed.

If high blood pressure continues to injure the arterial lining, a plaque develops, containing fibrous clot material and fats absorbed from the blood. This process illustrates clearly how many of the high risk factors co-ordinate to produce plaque disease.

While hypertension damages the arterial lining, high stress levels – themselves a major cause of hypertensive disease – release the hormones adrenaline and noradrenaline from the adrenal glands. High blood levels of these two chemicals in turn increase the blood's clotting tendency.

THE HUMAN ARTERY

In this context, the human artery itself is a hindrance rather than a help. It has been referred to as 'the worst made of all the mammals'.' A vital aspect of atherosclerosis is the poor perfusion of the arteries' smooth muscular wall by oxygen and nutrients. Deposition of a fibrous plaque on its inner wall further reduces its oxygen and nutrient supply.

The transport of molecules through the arterial wall is another important factor. Human arteries often have patches where permeability to these molecules is particularly high. This problem, intensified by hypertension and the ageing process, weakens the arteries' ability to combat thrombosis.

Atherosclerosis is linked in many ways with diet – a factor that will be discussed at length in Chapter 5. A point of relevance to atheromatous plaque development, though, should be mentioned here. The process may be made worse by an immunological reaction to foreign proteins. Dr David Davies, a pathologist at the West Wales General Hospital, Carmarthen, outlined a long-term study in the newspaper *Doctor* (13 October 1983). He pointed out that death from myocardial infarction (heart attack) was sometimes associated with the presence of antibodies to milk in the blood of the victims. Male patients were found to have a threefold chance of dying from a second or subsequent heart attack if milk antibodies were present at the time when the first one occurred. The mechanism was not clear, but simple experiments had shown that milk proteins can cause blood platelets to clump together as they do during the initial stage of clot formation.

At the time of this report, Dr Patrick Gallagher from Southampton General Hospital had shown in laboratory experiments that the ability to tolerate soya protein reduced the incidence of atheroma threefold, although he was unable to support Dr Davies' milk antibody findings.

London GP Dr Jeffry Segall suggested that lactose (i.e. milk sugar) may cause coronary heart disease. He pointed out the relatively high number of people (83–98 per cent) in North West Europe capable of absorbing this substance, compared with the figure in Japan (22 per cent) and in other regions where the incidence of deaths from coronary artery disease is low.

Coronary Heart Disease

The heart never ceases its work of pumping oxygenated blood into the arterial system. Its muscular walls get a few moments' respite during the diastolic (i.e. relaxation) phase between beats. Yet it contracts between 70 and 80 times per minute, day and night, for an average of 70 years and, in a few people, for as long as 100 years.

The walls of the heart consist of highly specialized muscular tissue of great durability and considerable strength, and in need of a constant and adequate oxygen supply. Other muscles are allowed to recover after exercise. If we are unfit and sprint a couple of hundred yards to catch a train or bus, the heart and lungs are unable to meet the sudden demand for extra oxygen-rich blood.

Our leg muscles are depleted of oxygen by the uncustomary activity and become painful, both on this account and because of the accumulation of waste products of metabolism (cellular activity). We are at liberty to rest them, though, until their supply of arterial blood is restored, the toxic chemicals are removed and the oxygen debt is repaid.

Unlike the calf muscles, the heart cannot rest after extra effort. It is, in fact, the source of its own blood supply! The coronary arteries bringing blood to its walls arise from the aorta, just as this vessel leaves the left side of the heart. The heart has to continue to pump in order for blood to flow along them and perfuse every area of its tissues. Coronary arteries narrowed by atheromatous plaques seriously limit cardiac (i.e. heart) function.

Angina

The chest pain that results from shortage of oxygen to the heart is a symptom about which a doctor should be consulted without delay. The pain can be intense, and may extend from the centre of the chest down one arm (generally the left) and up into the root of the neck. It can be triggered by sudden physical exertion, excitement, shock or emotional stress, and is an advance warning of a possible heart attack.

Unstable angina is angina arising when you are at rest, or with increasing frequency and severity. Once thought to be caused by coronary artery spasm intermittently disturbing arterial blood flow, it is now thought possibly to result from recurrent clot formation in the damaged area of a coronary artery.

In 1986, a Glasgow research team's paper in the *British Heart Journal* reported that squash players frequently continued with their sport despite being fully aware, having suffered attacks of angina, that the condition of their heart was inadequate to the demand. They had investigated 60 sudden deaths in the UK between 1976 and 1984, associated with squash. The victim's average age was 46 years, and ranged from 22 to 66. All were white, all but one were male, and the majority came from professional or executive families. Coronary artery disease accounted for 58 of the 60 deaths. All had many risk factors – *the commonest of which was hypertension*. Overall, 45 of the victims had reported signs of heart disease, nearly always angina.

Heart attacks resulting from coronary artery disease are the commonest cause of fatality in many strenuous sports. Deaths occurring during marathon running, soccer, rugby football, basketball and tennis have all been investigated. In one survey, they were responsible for 73 per cent of 109 deaths. Almost half of these occurred in men with well-documented risk factors, and one third had suffered from warning signs – known as 'prodromal symptoms' – such as extreme fatigue or anginal chest pain.

Experts urge all sports participants to seek medical attention for any untoward health problems, and evidence of damaged coronary arteries or impaired heart function means that they should stop playing that particular sport.

Heart Attacks

Heart attacks end or cripple the lives of sportsmen and many others with coronary heart disorder. Known medically as *myocardial infarction*, or simply 'MI', they are caused in nearly all cases by severe narrowing of a major coronary artery by atheromatous plaques, and the eventual obstruction of that artery by a tear in its lining or by a clot (i.e. coronary thrombosis). The area of heart muscle (myocardium) deprived of blood becomes 'infarcted', that is, it suffers irreversible damage due to oxygen and nutrient deprivation.

The extent of the myocardial infarct determines the severity of the heart attack: although massive ones usually kill, recovery following many is quite satisfactory, the damaged heart muscle undergoing repair by the formation of scar tissue.

Hypertension and a high blood fat (cholesterol) level are the two most important risk factors predisposing to atherosclerosis and heart attacks. Heart disease mortality figures are higher in the UK than anywhere else in the world, the worst 'death spots' being Wales, Scotland and Northern Ireland. Heart and circulatory disease kills more people in Britain than any other disorder, including all types of cancer grouped together, and claims one life every three minutes, i.e. 200,000 annually.

Changes in habit and attitude, a healthy diet and a sound strategy for normalizing blood pressure can do much to improve this dismal outlook. They have already been put into practice on a large scale in the USA, Australia, New Zealand and Canada: countries with lifestyles similar to the UK and with comparable past records of heart disease mortality rates.

The heart attack death rate has fallen in some of these countries by up to 37 per cent. In the UK it fell by 3 per cent in 1986 compared to that of the previous year, but the overall figures for the past 15 years show a 3 per cent rise in the death rate among men *and a 10 per cent rise in the death rate among women* although the introduction of blood clot-destroying agents such as streptokinase in the 1990s (and supplementary anti-clotting medication) has transformed the management of acute MI, and many more people now survive the initial attack and have better-functioning hearts, too, in the aftermath of the attack.

Before looking in detail at what can be done to improve the situation, we must place conventional medical treatment in its proper perspective. To do so, it is essential to understand its underlying rationale and the means by which antihypertensive drugs reduce and control high blood pressure, and this will be dealt with in the next chapter.

Chapter four

The Treatment Controversy

Since hypertension was first known to predispose sufferers to heart attacks and strokes, several conflicting viewpoints about its treatment have struggled for supremacy. It is easy for uninformed people to dismiss this state of affairs by quoting cynically that 'doctors differ and patients die'. Nevertheless, controversy about medical treatment, although in many ways less than satisfactory, is in fact a healthy sign. It means that a great deal of research attention is being directed towards solving a certain problem – in this case, finding out as much as possible about hypertension and hypertensive patients, and establishing the most effective and safest treatment method.

Inevitably, when various theories are put forward and tested and new drugs are developed, the pool of knowledge assumes a murky appearance, with so many doctors and scientists earnestly stirring the waters, hoping the answer will soon reach the surface! The patients involved in surveys and clinical trials show varying group profiles; and, although computers analyse trial data, human beings rather than machines interpret them.

The further research progresses, the more experts are coming to realize the true complexity of hypertensive disease. Research into the problem has produced impressive results over the past 15 years, and although much remains to be done, it should not be too long before the answers to many important questions become clear.

According to experts – cardiologists, epidemiologists (who study disease, populations and environment), physiologists, geneticists – speaking at the International Society of Hypertension (ISH) biennial meeting held in the summer of 1988, hypertension cannot be considered a single entity. It is now recognized as a final common pathway through which a number of complex and abnormal physiological processes – metabolic, genetic, environmental – manifest themselves. The fact that numerous possible causes exist explains why no single antihypertensive drug, or group of drugs, treats all sufferers satisfactorily. It also complicates treatment.

MILD AND MODERATE HYPERTENSION

Mildly hypertensive people (i.e. those with a diastolic blood pressure between 95 and 105 mm Hg – *see Chapter 2*) were once considered better off without medication, at least initially. Speaking at an international symposium on hypertension in New Orleans in 1983, Professor Norman Kaplan from the University of Texas said that patients within this category had a low mortality, and that only three out of every thousand patients would benefit from medication. He pointed out that if drug therapy were withheld the blood pressure would fall spontaneously to below 90 mm Hg in about one-third of these patients.

Interestingly, he suggested lifestyle changes, including weight loss where appropriate, as the preferred approach, and drugs as a last resort only if the blood pressure remained above 100 mm Hg after six months.

Opinions remained divided on this issue for some time. The aim of treating hypertension is to reduce the incidence of angina, heart attacks and other disorders discussed in the previous chapter. The rationale of treating mild to moderate degree of hypertension did not start to become established until the early 1970s when a wide choice of antihypertensive drugs started to appear.

A series of long-term studies reported in the *Journal of the American Medical Association* in April 1988 produced scientific evidence of a valuable reduction in deaths in such patients from coronary heart disease as well as from strokes, heart failure and kidney disease. A total of 3,234 male patients suffering from mild to moderate hypertension were treated in this research trial, known as the MAPHY study (primary prevention with metoprolol in patients with hypertension), either with a thiadize diuretic drug or with the beta blocker metoprolol (Betaloc, Lopressor).

They were followed up clinically for an average of 4.16 years; the reduction in blood pressure was equal in both treatment groups but there were significantly fewer deaths from heart attacks and strokes among those patients given the beta blocker.

WOMEN AND HYPERTENSION

The treatment of women with high blood pressure is given special consideration in many reports. Some research trials have indicated that women with mild to moderate hypertension benefit less than men from drug therapy. In one study conducted by the British Medical Research Council which included 9,048 men and 8,306 women aged 35 to 64 years, the patients were treated with either a placebo (dummy) and diuretic, or a beta blocker drug, and were followed up for 5½ years.

The rate of strokes and cardiovascular problems fell significantly in both sexes, and response to drug treatment was similar in a number of ways. However, while the overall death rate was reduced among male patients by active treatment, it was increased among females (but see the Amery study mentioned below).

Reasons for the latter finding may include increases in the consumption of alcohol and in smoking by women. Both increase the risks of high blood pressure, and so does obesity. Women who drink more than the recommended amount (*see Chapter 9*) and/or quit smoking tend to put on more weight than men — one study showed an average gain of 21 lb

(10 kg) in women who had abandoned cigarettes. This is a major deterrent to would-be non-smokers, and emphasizes the need for a healthy, calorie-controlled diet and exercise to combat overweight (see Chapter 5).

THE ELDERLY AND HYPERTENSION

There is now substantial evidence that active treatment of mild to moderate hypertension in elderly people reduces the risks of associated ill-health and death. The Veterans Administration (VA) studies of 1967, 1970 and 1972, which were confined to males, suggested that the elderly derived the same benefits from blood pressure reductions as younger individuals.

The Australian study of mild to moderate hypertension (National Heart Foundation of Australia, 1981) backed this finding in their male participants, and the 1985 European study carried out by A. Amery and colleagues and reported in *The Lancet* showed unequivocally that treatment benefited elderly patients. It reduced cardiovascular deaths by 37 per cent in those with a diastolic pressure of 90–99 mm Hg, and by 50 per cent in those with a diastolic reading between 100–119 mm Hg *in both sexes*.

More recently (1993), the British Hypertension Society published its guidelines in the *British Medical Journal* advising that patients *under 60* should definitely be treated if their diastolic pressure levels were at 100 mm Hg or more; and that patients over 60 should definitely receive treatment for a systolic pressure of 160 mm Hg or more; a diastolic pressure of 90 mm Hg or more; or both. Some studies in Sweden (1991), the US (1991) and Britain (Medical Research Council, 1992) have found that very elderly patients (over 80 years) benefit from treatment *at least* until the age of 86, if not over.

CHOICE OF MEDICATION

Malignant Hypertension

Malignant or 'accelerated' hypertension is a medical emergency requiring immediate treatment. The diastolic pressure is frequently in the range of 130 to 170 mm Hg, and the patient often feels very ill, with common symptoms including headaches, giddy spells, blackouts, breathlessness and blurred vision.

The retina of the eye is damaged and the optic nerve disc is swollen (papilloedema). This the physician detects by examining the retina through the pupil of the eye with a lighted instrument (ophthalmoscope) in a suitably darkened room.

There may be evidence of kidney or heart disease, and hypertensive encephalophy – generalized brain swelling due to leakage of blood plasma through the walls of damaged brain arterioles – is another serious complication.

Most patients with malignant hypertension are hospitalized at once. Gravely ill patients requiring immediate blood pressure reduction may receive an intravenous injection or drip infusion of labetolol (Trandate), a combined alpha and beta blocker (*see below*). The rate of administration is carefully monitored because it is dangerous to reduce the blood pressure too rapidly.

'Stepped Care' Treatment

The 'stepped care' method of treating all patients with mild to moderate hypertension emerged in the early 1970s, and provided doctors with a sequence of therapeutic manoeuvres which would ensure the reduction of blood pressure to a satisfactory level. Step 1 was generally a diuretic at less than full dose, step 2 was the diuretic at full dose and step 3 was the addition of methyldopa, reserpine or a beta blocker. If control remained

Step 0 Non-pharmacological treatment
Step 1 Thiazide *or* beta blocker
Step 2 Thiazide *and* beta blocker
Step 3 Thiazide *and* beta blocker *and* vasodilator
Step 4 Resistant hypertension regimens

Fig. 3 'Stepped care' treatment

unsatisfactory, further drugs were added or substituted until the desirable blood pressure was achieved – see Fig. 3.

As W. A. Littler, Professor of Cardiovascular Medicine at the University of Birmingham, points out in *Cardiovascular Focus 22*, Bayer UK Ltd, the success of any regimen depends ultimately upon patients' compliance; 50 per cent of patients with symptoms and 60 per cent of patients without symptoms do not take the drugs as directed. The simpler the treatment, the more likely the patient will be to remain on therapy and take it as prescribed.

As new antihypertensive drugs were developed, the original stepped care scheme underwent several changes, with vasodilator drugs such as hydralazine (Apresoline) replacing those at step 3. By the end of 1985, the massive amount of information that had been obtained from trials and studies on hypertensive treatment placed stepped care policy under careful scrutiny. Today's approach is far broader, and its most interesting aspect is step 0, which refers to natural blood pressure control methods.

Professor Littler (and many other experts) now feel that a more individualized approach to hypertensive patients should be adopted in preference to a 'slavish pursuit of a prescribed regimen'. He advocates *more non-pharmacological (i.e. natural) techniques for the management of mild hypertension*, and emphasizes that the patient's quality of life must always be borne in mind.

Clinical studies have shown that the more recently introduced drugs – alpha blockers, combined alpha-beta blockers, calcium antagonists and ACE inhibitors – are as effective at controlling blood pressure as many of the older ones. Initially they were assigned to steps 3 and 4 in the stepped care programme, but calcium antagonists and ACE inhibitors are now considered much earlier on: they can be used alone, together, or with diuretics or beta blockers, and are thought to have advantages over these last two traditional standbys.

Doses of all drugs are now kept as low as possible and given in time-release form wherever possible. This allows a once-daily dose to be taken.

PATIENTS, DOCTORS AND MEDICATION

Few patients are told enough about the medication they are expected to take. Certainly no doctor can be expected to give each patient a mini-lecture in physiology and pharmacology; but at least people need to be told which drugs are being prescribed for their condition, what these drugs can be expected to do, and possible side-effects to watch out for.

Consultation time during busy surgeries does make this difficult; and some doctors understandably object to reeling off lists of side-effects to their patients, on the grounds that the power of suggestion alone can produce an impressive display of symptoms in anxious, stressed, highly imaginative people. The solution is, of course, to explain just what is necessary, avoiding over-lavish discussions of adverse reactions which, although described in the drug literature, are frequently very rare.

It is only when doctors co-operate with patients and treat them as intelligent human beings that compliance with medication regimens can be expected to improve. It is also the only sure way to convince hypertensive patients who feel perfectly fit of the necessity of following medical advice.

How Antihypertensive Drugs Work

Here, then, is how the main groups of antihypertensive drugs go about reducing blood pressure. Skip this section if you prefer; but becoming more familiar with whatever medication you are presently taking may encourage you to take it as prescribed, and/or make you determined to set complementary self-help methods into operation from this moment onwards!

Most antihypertensive drugs work in highly complex ways. The following is a brief and highly simplified summary of how the most important ones reduce blood pressure.

Diuretics act on the kidney tubules and cause sodium and water excretion, thereby reducing the volumes of the blood plasma and the extracellular fluid bathing the tissue cells. Extra urine is passed, the pressure due to constricted arterioles is lowered, the strain on the heart is reduced and the blood pressure falls. Low doses of diuretics work as well as high doses and produce fewer side-effects.

Black people generally respond better to diuretics than to beta blockers as initial treatment for hypertension, and a diuretic is therefore usually chosen for treating them unless there are contra-indications to its use.

Beta blockers, properly called 'beta-adrenergic blocking agents', counteract the blood pressure-raising effects of noradrenaline produced by the adrenal glands. They compete with this stress hormone for action upon highly specialized 'beta-adrenergic receptor cells' which play significant roles in the control of blood pressure. Highly responsive to noradrenaline, which increases blood pressure, these cells are widely distributed throughout the body, and are found in particularly large numbers in the heart, lungs and blood vessels.

The explanation of precisely how these drugs lower blood pressure is poorly understood, but it is thought that the heart's output of blood (cardiac output) is reduced without the usual compensatory 'clamping down' of the arterioles. In addition, the kidneys release less renin and this also causes blood pressure to fall.

Although they lower the 'useful' type of blood cholesterol (the high-density variety) and are unsuitable for asthmatics and people with defects in the heart's electrical conducting system, beta blockers are currently preferred by many doctors for step 1 therapy in white people, especially in cases where diuretic drugs are inappropriate.

Vasodilators – since the main problem in hypertension is increased resistance to blood flow because of constricted arterioles, the use of drugs that directly dilate arterial vessels seems the most logical approach to treatment. (This is a point which illustrates the scientific approach of allopathic medicine. Holistic – i.e. alternative – practitioners would strongly disagree, pointing out that tight-walled arterioles are in fact a *symptom* of a deeper, more complex problem affecting the entire person. However, here we are considering how orthodox medicines work and the reasoning – valid according to its own underlying premises – of how the particular illness in question arises.)

Vasodilator drugs have a relaxing effect upon the smooth muscle of the arteriolar walls. This lessens peripheral resistance and lowers the blood pressure. Hydralazine (Apresoline) becomes tightly bound to the blood vessel walls and acts for longer than some of the others. Vasodilator therapy is used in combination with a beta blocker and diuretic to treat moderate to severe hypertension.

Calcium antagonists, like vasodilators, lower resistance and blood pressure by relaxing constricted arterioles. Their action relies upon inhibiting the passage of calcium ions (electrically charged calcium atoms) into the smooth muscle walls.

They can be used alone (*see above*); or nifedipine (Adalat) and nicardipine (Cardene) may be prescribed together with beta blockers. They are useful for patients suffering from diseased arteries of the lower limbs; and for asthmatics, for whom beta blockers are generally unsuitable.

ACE (angiotensin-converting enzyme) inhibitors work by combating the action of the enzyme responsible for converting the relatively inactive substance angiotensin I into its more potent form, angiotensin II. The latter triggers the production and secretion of aldosterone, a hormone manufactured in the centre of the adrenal glands, which acts powerfully on the arteriolar walls, constricting them and raising the blood pressure.

ACE inhibitors lower both diastolic and systolic pressure in all grades of hypertension, maintain the blood flow in the blood vessels of both brain and heart, and rarely cause postural hypotension. They provide valuable treatment for heart failure and damaged heart muscle (myocardial infarction) and reduce the formation of fibrous tissue (which interferes with the heart's pumping action) after an MI. They also have a beneficial effect upon the kidneys and increase urine production, thereby reducing the load upon a damaged or labouring heart. Unlike beta blockers, they are safe for both asthmatics and diabetics. They do not affect cholesterol blood levels, and neither deplete the body's potassium stores nor predispose it to gout or to hyperglycaemia (raised blood sugar levels – the diabetes problem).

Patients taking ACE inhibitors seldom complain of adverse effects. They are effective in all grades of hypertension, including severe forms which have failed to respond to other forms of treatment.

Alpha blockers counteract the constrictive effects of noradrenaline upon the arterioles by competing for attachment to alpha-receptor cells in the walls of these vessels. They are especially useful for controlling hypertension associated with excessive amounts of adrenaline and noradrenaline in the blood.

Combined alpha and beta blockers control blood pressure by alpha effects and by concurrent beta effects (*see above*) upon the heart. The systolic blood pressure rise that normally accompanies exercise is reduced, although the diastolic rise remains the same as usual. Drugs of this type benefit hypertensive patients with co-existing angina, and are suitable for treating hypertension of all degrees of severity.

Part two

Reducing Your Blood Pressure Naturally

Chapter five

Diet and Weight Control

On 18 January 1986, the weekly GPs' newsletter *Pulse* published an article entitled: 'Hypertension: Which Drug For Which Patient?' by Dr Richard Pearson, consultant physician at St Bartholomew's Hospital, London. In it, he commented:

> Recently, there has been immense interest in the use of non-drug treatments as adjuncts or *alternatives* [my italics] to drug therapy. A wide range of interventions has been shown to reduce raised blood pressure, but not all have been shown to reduce its complications.
>
> Following this advice will often allow patients to be treated with smaller doses of drugs than they would otherwise need. This will lead to better tolerated treatment, better compliance and better control but it is unlikely to obviate the need for drugs in most cases.

The writer is being wisely cautious. Many patients with moderate to severe hypertension, especially when it has been long established (as well as a few with the mild variety), *do* require continuous medication. If this turns out to be true in your case, be cheered by the prospect of reducing the doses of drugs you are taking, and thereby any side-effects you may experience.

Remember, too, that hypertension is a highly complex condition, and that each hypertensive patient is an individual with his or her own built-in capacity to respond to natural therapy. It may seem unlikely, for a variety of reasons, that *you* will be able to stop medication altogether. But natural treatment frequently produces unexpected improvements, and will certainly increase your general health.

Regarding the effects of natural treatment on the complications of hypertension, this must depend upon the severity and duration of the problems involved. Successful blood pressure reduction relieves the strain on the heart, and a mild degree of failure is reversible. Serious damage to kidney, eye (*see malignant hypertension in Chapter 4*) or brain is beyond the scope of most experts, orthodox or complementary, to reverse.

Dr Pearson goes on to comment upon the benefits of weight loss, exercise, relaxation, ceasing to smoke and reducing alcohol intake, and states: 'Dietary modifications have been widely advised and are generally accepted.'

DIET: ITS AIMS

The word 'diet' has a doleful ring. Litanies are sung in the praise of every one invented, yet disillusion invariably sets in if they are regimentally organized and too demanding. Perhaps diets, as popularly interpreted, are the one health control method the majority of people are eager to try, and the one most often abandoned as unsuccessful and depressing.

'Dietary modifications' sounds even worse. This usually refers to a restricted eating pattern designed for weight reduction, or the control of diabetes or some other illness. The dictionary definition of diet, however, puts the matter into a welcome perspective. It is, simply, 'the usual food and drink of a person or animal'. So we will continue to use this convenient shorthand term for a way of eating that is 'modified' with four main aims in view. These are:

1. to improve general health, increase vitality and boost energy
2. to reduce high blood pressure
3. to reduce a high serum cholesterol level
4. to reduce and stabilize body weight.

While the first two will apply to you if you suffer from high blood pressure, the last two may not. We did see in the last chapter, though, that in Britain the *average* serum cholesterol tends to be way above that of other populations with a low incidence of heart disease; so there is every reason to keep a careful check on your own levels.

Similarly your weight may be ideal, or even on the low side, for your height and build (notice that I do not mention age – we will look at this in more detail in the final section). You are to be envied or congratulated, depending upon your metabolism or your self-control! A millennium study commissioned by the Bread for Life organization indicated that obesity has reached epidemic proportions in the UK, with 17 per cent of men and 20 per cent of women being obese, and more than 50 per cent of the population overweight. If present trends continue, more than 25 per cent of the UK population will be obese by 2010

You may eat normally and have no need to count calories. If you maintain your normal-to-low weight by stringent diets, however, you will be able to reject these time-wasters in favour of a healthier and more acceptable eating pattern that will control your weight naturally.

Whole Foods and Public Attitude

Whole foods are the subject of as much controversy among the population at large as aspects of hypertensive treatment are among doctors!

Support for natural foods is growing. Consumption of full-cream dairy products, white bread, red meat and eggs has fallen, and demand for wholemeal bread, low-fat sausages, skimmed milk and reduced-fat dairy products, and fresh fruit and vegetables has increased. This trend must partly account for the slight decline in the gradient of the heart attack death rate which, in 1986, had dropped by 3 per cent compared with 1985.

You may already be a whole food enthusiast. Some people, however, detest the term, relegating it to a minority of health cranks with plenty of time to follow weird recipes and ample cash to spend on ingredients.

'Anti whole fooders' see no point in altering their usual diet, and continue to relish their fish and chips, chocolate bars, commercial ice cream and sliced white bread. They maintain that no one in the family will eat wholemeal bread, and that it goes off quickly; that raw fruit takes too long to chew when a quick snack is needed; that the fresh vegetables need preparation and longer cooking time than their frozen or canned equivalents; and that life is not worth living without food you can look forward to and enjoy!

The inappropriate moral attitude that some whole food enthusiasts, in common with many non-smokers, have assumed is partly responsible for this reaction. Health zealots, among them certain food manufacturers who make 'additive absence' their selling point, dogmatize what is no more than a sane and practical way of eating.

Smug proselytizing is useless – and may endanger the nation's health! It reinforces people's determination to carry on as before. Assertive types condemn all health advice as rubbish, while the more timid, equally determined not to be dictated to, simply dive underground, taking their habits with them!

Sensitive smokers in small communities have been known to whisper a request for 20 of their favourite brand at supermarket checkouts, hoping no one in the queue behind will notice the transaction! This is how embarrassed young girls often behaved in the 1950s when buying a packet of 'STs' (sanitary towels)! At this rate, the courageous purchasers of sliced white bread will soon be burying their loaves at the bottom of their baskets, and smuggling them out via the fire exit!

Whole food eating is not a religion. It ordains neither priests nor preachers, and promises no health paradise for those who keep its commandments! But you'll follow its guidelines *if* you are convinced the results will be worthwhile. A whole food diet, together with other measures, will increase your energy and resistance to illness, and help to reduce your blood pressure. You may even find it brings an end to bimonthly prescriptions for antihypertensive drugs!

What are Whole Foods?

They are foods to which nothing has been added, and from which nothing has been removed. They are *the* foods for everyone who desires to remain or to become as healthy as possible. They are collectively the natural human diet, unimpoverished by efforts to improve their colour, flavour, texture and durability. And they are superabundantly rich in the nutrients – vitamins, minerals, trace elements, fibre and amino acids – essential to human biochemistry.

Research has produced a score of international reports recommending changes in our present way of eating, and emphasizing the dietary significance of whole foods. Two British Government reports, NACNE (the National Advisory Council on Nutrition Education) and COMA (Committee on the Medical Aspects of Food Policy) have agreed the findings. Further studies have shown that whole foods guard against obesity, stomach and bowel disease, allergies, depression, chronic fatigue, certain cancers, diabetes and many other disorders, and can help to relieve them once they have developed. They are highly beneficial to the circulatory system, and therefore to people suffering from high blood pressure.

Up to and including the first decades of the 20th century, everyone ate whole foods because there was nothing else! Wholemeal bread; fresh meat, poultry, fish and eggs; milk, butter and cheese; vegetables and fruit were everyday fare, and the food with which our grandparents and great-grandparents were familiar throughout their lives.

Far from today's technology improving the flavour of real food, it is far more apt to destroy it. Elderly people today who remember a different era are correct when they claim that food today does not taste as it once did. Battery egg production, crop pesticide sprays, the hormone treatment of farm animals and food processing techniques are among the many factors that impair the flavour, texture and nutritional value of the modern diet.

Certainly malnutrition was a grave problem in past times for the underprivileged. Epidemics of infectious illness caused many more fatalities than they would today, and rickets (a bone disease caused by vitamin D deficiency) was rife among poor children during the Industrial Revolution.

Of greater relevance here, however, is the fact that heart disease was virtually unknown at the turn of the century. Canadian Baronet Sir William Osler, probably the most brilliant physician of his time (1849–1919), admitted that he would find the condition harder to diagnose than many others, since he had seen no more than a small handful of cases throughout the whole of his professional life. Controversy continues, however, over whether this was because heart disease actually affected far fewer people, or because knowledge of the condition was rudimentary compared to how much is known in the early 21st century, and fewer diagnoses of it were made.

Ironically, the problem of malnutrition is still with us. Much of what we eat is lacking in essential nutrients. We eat far more fat and sugar, about the same amount of protein, and far less natural carbohydrate. We eat fewer potatoes and less bread 'because they are fattening', less fibre and fewer grains, vegetables and fruit.

BLOOD PRESSURE AND DIET

Many aspects of our modern lifestyle can be held responsible for the present epidemic of coronary heart disease. Among them, our diet, especially with the ready availability of high fat and high sugar processed convenience foods, is considered by many health experts to be the chief culprit.

In 1999, a paper was published in the *American Archives of Internal Medicine* reporting the findings of DASH, a study of Dietary Approaches to Stop Hypertension supported by the National Heart, Lung and Blood Institute. Designed to test the effects of eating patterns on blood pressure, DASH enrolled 459 people – some with normal and others with raised blood pressure – willing to eat food provided by the organizers in place of their normal diet for 11 weeks. They also had to keep daily food diaries, and take their main meal five days a week at one of the four participating clinics.

The group, which had an average age of 44.6 years, included 49 per cent women and 59 per cent African Americans. Those being treated for high blood pressure had their medication withdrawn for the duration of the study and, to ensure that all the subjects started off on the same footing, they all consumed a 'typical American' diet for the first three weeks.

They were then assigned at random to one of three diets for the remaining eight weeks:

1. a continuation of the control diet
2. a similar diet, but enriched with fruit and vegetables
3. one both enriched with fruit, vegetables and low-fat dairy products, and reduced in saturated fats

Diet 2 supplied extra potassium and a variety of other minerals and vitamins present in fruit and vegetables, as well as extra fibre. Diet 3, dubbed the 'combination' diet because it brought together several features thought to lower blood pressure, offered the same benefits as diet 2, as well as extra calcium, magnesium, protein and fibre, and reduced intakes of total fat, saturated fat and cholesterol.

Factors which could affect the outcome, such as body weight, sodium intake and alcohol consumption, were taken into account. Calorie consumption was tailored to individual needs, where necessary, to maintain body weight; all three diets provided about 3000mg of sodium daily (about 20 per cent less than average intake); and volunteers maintained their usual level of alcohol consumption. Compliance with the diet was assessed from the food diaries, observation during the main meals at the study sites, and the excretion of key nutrients in 24-hour urine specimens. All three groups stuck to their assigned diets with equal success, and 'prescribed foods only' were consumed on 94 per cent of the days throughout the eight-week period.

Blood pressures were measured over five to seven different days, both at the beginning and at the end of the eight-week test period. The clinical staff involved with this were kept deliberately unaware of which diet each subject was following, to avoid any influence this knowledge might have on the readings. An average of these pre- and post-study readings was used to measure the effects of the diets.

The average BP at the start was 132/85, which matches 40 per cent of the adult US population. The following chart shows the reductions in systolic and diastolic values in millimetres of mercury after eight weeks on the three diets:

	Systolic	Diastolic	Number of volunteers
Control diet	−1.1	0.6	154
Fruit/veg diet	−3.9*	−1.7	154
Combination diet	−6.7*	−3.6*	151

* = Statistically significantly different from Control Diet.

As you can see, the fruit and vegetable-enriched diet reduced systolic pressure, while the combination diet had about double the influence, and reduced both systolic and diastolic pressure. The beneficial effect, which was apparent after one week, peaked at two weeks and remained stable from then on. Similar reductions were seen in men and women and, interestingly, the 133 people with raised blood pressure experienced a greater lowering effect than those with normal readings on the combination diet:

	Systolic pressure	Diastolic pressure
Normal blood pressure subjects	–3.5	–2.1
Raised blood pressure subjects	–11.4	–5.5

The DASH study examined eating patterns and whole foods, and it is not possible to deduce from it which dietary constituents actively reduce high BP. However, the average pressure reduction in the group of people with diagnosed high blood pressure was equivalent to that normally produced by a single antihypertensive drug (as opposed to combination therapy); and researchers have calculated that a population-wide blood pressure reduction like that seen in the DASH study would reduce coronary heart disease by 15 per cent and stroke by 27 per cent.

DASH researchers stated in their Study Rationale (the part of a study report explaining the reasoning on which the goal of the research is based) that they wished to examine the widely recognized efficacy of a vegetarian diet in lowering blood pressure, while including just enough animal protein to make it generally acceptable. Many studies have examined the role(s) of isolated constituents of vegetarian eating in a bid to identify the 'active' component, but little useful information has resulted. Potassium supplements have been found to reduce blood pressure to an extent, but magnesium and calcium supplements and changes in fat consumption have shown little benefit.

This does not mean that nutritional supplements have no part to play in the overall reduction and control of high blood pressure. We'll explore this role in a later chapter; meanwhile, we need to look at the food groups and daily serving sizes recommended in consequence of the DASH study.

Food group	Daily servings	Serving sizes	Examples	Benefits
Grains	7–8	1 slice bread, 1 cup cereal ¹/₂ cup cooked rice or pasta	bread: wholewheat, pumpernickel, light or dark rye; English muffin, crumpet, bagel, couscous, spaghetti	Energy and fibre
Vegetables	4–5	1 cup raw leafy veg, ¹/₂ cup cooked veg, 170ml (6fl oz) veg. juice	root veg, spinach, cauliflower, artichokes, sweet sweet potatoes, green beans	Potassium, magnesium, fibre, other minerals and vitamins
Fruit	4–5	170ml (6fl oz) fruit juice, 1 medium fruit ¹/₄ cup dried fruit 1¹/₂ cups frozen or canned fruit	pineapple juice, apple, pear slice of papaya (paw paw) or melon 2–3 greengages	Potassium, magnesium, fibre, other minerals and vitamins
Low-fat or fat-free dairy products	2–3	230ml (8fl oz) milk, 1 cup yogurt 30–55g (1–2oz) cheese	low- or no-fat milk, fromage frais, crème fraîche yoghurt; cottage cheese, other medium or reduced fat hard cheese	Calcium and protein
Meat, fish, poultry	2 or fewer	85–115g (3–4oz) cooked meat, poultry or fish	lamb's liver, steak, cod, plaice, chicken	Protein and magnesium
Nuts, seeds, dried pulses	4–5 a week	15g (¹/₂oz) nuts, 2 tbsp seeds, ¹/₂ cup cooked dried beans	cashews, walnuts, pumpkin seeds, flageolet or haricot beans	Energy, potassium, magnesium, protein and fibre

Food group	Daily servings	Serving sizes	Examples	Benefits
Fats and oils	2–3	1 tbsp soft margarine, 1 tsp vegetable oil	olive oil, low-fat spray-on vegetable oil, 1 tbsp low-fat mayonnaise, 2 tbsp light salad dressing	Energy and essential fatty acids necessary for a healthy heart and blood vessels and many body functions

My Tips On Taking Advantage of DASH

- Limit your sugar intake to 5-7 portions weekly – e.g. 1 tbsp sugar or golden syrup, 3 tsp jam or marmalade, 15g ($^1/_2$oz) sweets, 230ml (8fl oz) soft drink.
- Check your current diet – the changes you need to make may not be many.
- Introduce any you do need, one at a time, over a period of weeks.
- If the above table and the seven-day eating plan below strike you as spartan, remember the huge health benefits. They also provide a healthy foundation for safe weight loss so, if you want to shed a few kilos, customize the plan by adjusting the amounts and filling up on fresh raw or lightly cooked vegetables and fruit. You will then be truly thrilled with the diet, and thoroughly deserve to treat yourself to some favourite foods on special occasions.

SEVEN-DAY EATING PLAN

I have devised a seven-day eating plan based on the DASH chart, with a few modifications.

- The DASH chart doesn't mention eggs; 2–3 weekly are fine.
- I haven't specified low-fat or wholemeal/whole grain/'lean only' items in the recipes as I assume you are choosing the foods from the DASH chart. The same goes for portion sizes, e.g. for bread, fruit and vegetables, cereal etc.
- The quantities I give in the recipes are for four servings unless stated otherwise.
- I use the term 'seasoning' rather than salt and pepper to minimize sodium intake, so either give salt a miss or use a potassium-based substitute.
- I use fresh herbs wherever possible – use $1/2$ teaspoon measures of the dried equivalents if you prefer.
- Give wholemeal pasta a try – it is more filling and richer in vitamins and minerals than the refined sort, but does not supply more calories, weight for weight. My cooking times for pasta are based on the wholemeal variety, which takes about twice as long to cook.

Breakfast Daily

Fruit or vegetable juice or fresh fruit
Cereal with milk
Egg or portion of fish
Bread/toast with margarine and jam or marmalade
Beverages – tea, coffee (decaff if you have a heart problem), skimmed milk, water, diet sodas

Snacks

Choose fresh or dried fruit, fresh vegetable sticks, nuts, seeds, unsweetened popcorn, unsalted pretzels.

Day 1

LUNCH
Tuna (tinned in spring water) mashed with capers, a spot of Worcestershire sauce and the pulp of half a tomato, chopped. Eat on fresh light or dark rye bread, with roughly chopped, very crisp lettuce dressed with a little lemon juice and pepper.
Plain yoghurt mixed with a little runny or comb honey.

DINNER
Vegetarian or very low-fat sausages, potatoes boiled and mashed with a little skimmed milk and pepper, fresh or tinned tomatoes and fresh or frozen peas.

Gooseberry Fool
This healthy alternative to fool made with double cream is brimful of vitamins, minerals and fibre without the high fat and energy content.

455g (1 lb/3¼ cups) fresh gooseberries, topped and tailed
artificial sweetener
450–570ml (16–20fl oz/2–2½ cups) thick plain yoghurt or half yoghurt/ half fromage frais, chilled

1. Cook the gooseberries until soft in a little water, and sweeten. Chill, then drain off juice and set aside.

2. Fold the gooseberries gently into the yoghurt or yoghurt/fromage frais mixture, adding just enough juice to achieve the consistency of whipped cream.

Day 2

LUNCH
Egg and cress sandwich with tbsp mayonnaise and black pepper.
Plain or fruit yoghurt with 2 passion fruit.

DINNER
Perfect Plaice
Buy the freshest fish you can find – feel the healthy, colourless slime over the surface (if you get the chance!), and look for bright orange spots against a dark brown background. Any flat white fish can be used, but this method brings out the delicate plaice flavour particularly well. It could not be simpler.

1 medium plaice on the bone or 2 small fillets per person
3–4 tbsp water

1. Lay the fish on a microwaveable plate, pour over the water and cover.
2. Microwave on medium for 3–6 minutes, depending on your oven and the thickness of the fish.
3. Turn a whole fish over, half way through.
4. It is perfectly cooked when the plaice's translucent flesh has just turned opaque and is exuding the most delectable curdy white juice.
5. Serve with fresh spinach and olive and onion potatoes (see following instructions).

Fresh Spinach
Again, this could not be simpler.

115–225g (4–8oz/2–4 cups) fresh spinach per person
seasoning
a little crushed garlic and squeeze of lemon juice (optional)

1. Wash the spinach and shake over the sink to remove most of the water (there's no need to tear off the stalks).
2. Stuff into a saucepan, season, cover and cook over a medium heat, stirring from time to time to prevent it sticking.
3. When it starts to wilt, cut through roughly with a knife and replace lid. Continue cooking until greatly reduced in volume and a uniform dark green.
4. Strain thoroughly, squeezing out the water with the back of a spoon. Return to pan and stir in a little crushed garlic and a squeeze of lemon juice, if liked, and serve.

Olive and Onion Potatoes
1 large baking potato per person
Skimmed milk
Bunch of spring onions (scallions), trimmed and chopped
Black or green olives, rinsed, stoned and chopped

1. Wash the potato, pat dry and score all the way round the middle with a sharp knife.
2. Bake in a hot oven (450°F/230°C/gas mark 8) for 1 hour or until tender.
3. Cut round the score marks and separate, scoop out the potato flesh and mash with a just enough skimmed milk to achieve the consistency you like.
4. Mix in the chopped onions and olives, and pile back into the shells. Brown under the grill

5.   Eat the beautifully crisp potato skins (which you do not get with microwave cooking) spread with some of your daily margarine allowance or some very cold fromage frais.

Apricots Duchess of Malfi

Hunza apricots, imported from India and Afghanistan, are delicious. They originated in the Hunza valley where the people are noted for their longevity. Sun-dried, with their stones intact, they need to be soaked in cold water for several hours or overnight to release their delicious natural sweetness, then stewed gently as described below. You will find them in (some) health food stores.

455–565g (16–20oz/4–5 cups) fresh apricots or
115–170g (4–6oz) Hunza apricots or
1 large tin apricots in juice
poppy seeds, to serve

1.   For fresh apricots, use ripe fruit only, cover with water and stew gently until soft.
2.   Put either type of apricot when cooked, or the tinned variety, through a sieve, after removing the stones.
3.   Mix in just enough juice to make a meltingly smooth purée, and chill thoroughly.
4.   Scatter with poppy seeds and eat alone or with a little plain yoghurt.

Day 3

LUNCH
Fresh whelks, cockles or winkles in shells
A little malt vinegar or lemon juice
Seasoning
A hunk of fresh bread

Do not despise these little creatures from the deep. They or their relations may be eaten worldwide, but there is something quintessentially English about enjoying them for lunch with a dab of malt vinegar, pepper, bread and butter. (Cockles and mussels in little bottles of vinegar or brine are no substitute for this fresh feast.)

Peach or nectarine

DINNER
Half a grapefruit

Clovelly Chicken
There is no need to peel any of these vegetables – just scrub clean and chop. The combined smell of chicken and vegetables is utterly seductive, and the broth is to die for!

1 medium fresh or frozen chicken, thawed
6-8 cloves
1 large onion, cut into quarters or eighths
2-3 carrots, chopped
$1/4$ swede, cut into chunks
2–3 parsnips, depending on size, cut into chunks
2–3 small turnips, cut into chunks
seasoning
$1/2$ teaspoon mixed herbs

1. Wipe chicken inside and out with a damp cloth.
2. Bash the heads of the cloves and insert them into the onion chunks by their stalks.
3. Put onion pieces at the bottom of a large saucepan together with a few pieces of carrot, then place the bird on top. Fit all the other vegetable chunks in and around the chicken, season well, add the mixed

herbs and just cover with water. Heat quickly to boiling, skim off
any debris, then turn down the heat and just simmer for $2^1/_2$–3
hours – until the meat is falling off the bones (i.e. the longer
and slower, the better). You may need to top up with water once
or twice.

4.   Serve with some plain boiled potatoes and a bright green veg –
     Brussels sprouts, spinach or broccoli all hit the spot.

Baked Custard
3 medium free-range eggs
570ml (1 pint/$2^1/_2$ cups) reduced-fat milk
1–2 tbsp sugar
a few drops real vanilla or almond essence, if liked.

1.   Beat the eggs into the warmed milk, add sugar and essence, and
     strain into an ovenproof dish.
2.   Place the dish in a baking tin containing half an inch of cold water
     and bake in a moderate oven (325°F/170°C/gas mark 3) until set.
3.   Serve hot, tepid or cold, perhaps with a little stewed fresh fruit.

Day 4

LUNCH
Chicken and salad sandwich, with mayonnaise or dressing, if liked.

Ripe pear or three greengages/plums.

DINNER
Spaghetti with Tomato and Mushroom Sauce
225g (8oz) spaghetti
2 tsp olive oil

1 medium onion, finely sliced
1 clove of garlic, crushed or finely chopped
170g (6oz/1½ cups) button or field mushrooms, chopped
5–6 large tomatoes or medium/large can peeled tomatoes, roughly chopped
1 dessertspoon fresh basil, chopped
seasoning
115g (4oz/1 cup) cheese, grated

1. Cook spaghetti in boiling water until *al dente* (soft, but with a bit of bite) – about 10–15 minutes.
2. Heat olive oil in a medium saucepan, add onions and garlic, stir to coat with oil, cover and continue cooking over a low heat until soft (using this small quantity of oil allows the onion and garlic to stew in their own juices).
3. Add the mushrooms and tomatoes (with juice if using tinned, or enough boiling water to prevent sticking), and cook for 5–7 minutes over a medium heat, stirring until soft.
4. Add basil and seasoning, stir well and pour over drained spaghetti.
5. Serve cheese separately, or scatter over the top and brown under grill.

Nutty Pineapple

Most pistachios are sold salted in their partially opened shells. As a perfectionist you will doubtless rinse off the salt. Even so, a certain saltiness will linger, providing a pleasing contrast with the sweetness of the fruit, just as the chilled yoghurt does with the heated pineapple.

1–2 heaped tbsp thick plain yoghurt
Large slice of fresh or tinned pineapple
1 dessertspoon chopped pistachio nuts

1. Chill yoghurt for at least 2 hours.
2. Heat tinned pineapple in juice or fresh pineapple in a very little water, top with cold yoghurt and scatter with chopped pistachios.

Day 5

LUNCH
Clear Vegetable Broth with Toast Croutons
It is worth the trouble of chopping and slicing the vegetables finely (especially the onion) to ensure swift and even cooking.

1 stick celery, finely chopped
1 large carrot, finely chopped
1 onion or leek, finely sliced
handful of fresh or frozen peas or beans
2 bay leaves
seasoning
1 litre (1³/₄ pints) vegetable stock or water
slice of bread, toasted

1. Put all vegetables in a large pot with the bay leaves and seasoning, and cover with water (the addition of a few tbsp jellied stock, like that produced by Clovelly Chicken, greatly enhances the flavour).
2. Bring to the boil, reduce the heat and simmer for 15–20 minutes until the vegetables are tender.
3. Toast the bread, cut into small crouton squares and serve with the soup.

DINNER
Pork Fillet
Allow 115–170g (4–6oz) fresh pork fillet per person.

1.   Wipe fillet with a clean damp cloth, moisten both surfaces with a little fresh lemon juice and lay some fresh rosemary twigs along its upper surface.
2.   Wrap carefully in cooking foil and cook in a medium oven for 25 minutes to the pound (455g).
3.   Check the flesh is white i.e. cooked all the way through by making a small cut with a sharp knife before serving with boiled or tinned new potatoes, carrots, mashed swede and Caraway Cabbage (*see below*).

Caraway Cabbage

Anyone who likes caraway seeds will be converted to cabbage by this recipe, especially if you select a dew-fresh, bright-green specimen with tightly curled leaves and no discernible smell.

2 tsp olive oil
1 large onion, sliced
1 medium head very fresh white or green cabbage, roughly chopped
1-2 tsp caraway seeds
freshly ground black pepper

1.   Heat the olive oil then add the sliced onion, covering and cooking over a low to medium heat until soft but not browned.
2.   Add the cabbage, wet from its washing but not swamped, mixing it in with the onion and packing it down before covering tightly.
3.   Continue cooking over a low to medium heat for 5 minutes, add the caraway seeds and a good grinding of black pepper, and cook, covered, until soft and juicy throughout, with a lingering bite.

Orange Hotspur

Allow per person:
1 whole orange, peeled and finely sliced
2–3 tbsp fromage frais, well-chilled

1 level dessertspoon demerara sugar
1 tsp Curacao or Grand Marnier

1.   Place sliced orange in a small heatproof dish, top with the fromage frais and sprinkle with brown sugar.
2.   Flash under very hot grill until sugar melts. N.B. Don't turn your back for a second – it's a terror for burning!
3.   Pour over the liqueur and serve at once.

Day 6

LUNCH
Large salad using as many fresh and lightly cooked cold vegetables as possible.
Light salad dressing.
Wholemeal roll.
Large slice of papaya (pawpaw) or other exotic fruit.

DINNER
Dry-fried Steak and Chips
It really is easy to cook steak and chips with the minimum of fat. If you really love steak, buy the best organic fillet you can from a private supplier.

Allow per person:
1–2 tsp olive oil or other cooking oil
115–170g (4–6oz) frying steak
1–2 medium potatoes, halved

1.   Heat oil a non-stick frying pan over a medium heat, smearing it around with the back of a spoon to make it go as far as possible. Have steak ready, and add to pan when the latter is very hot.

2. For 3cm ($1^{1}/_{2}$-inch) thickness, cook $1^{1}/_{2}$ minutes each side for blue/rare, $2^{1}/_{2}$–3 minutes a side for medium, and $3^{1}/_{2}$–4 minutes a side for well done. You will have to reduce the heat slightly for the longer cooking times to avoid burning. (Note: eating meat that is not cooked through carries the (slight) risk of food poisoning. Cook thoroughly, therefore, if you are elderly, in poor health or pregnant.)
3. Eat your steak with carrots, mushrooms, broad beans and chips.

Fatless Potato Chips
Microwave fatless chip devices into which you insert sliced raw potato and cook on high power, have never worked for me. Despite following the instructions, nothing happened at all – the 'chips' did not even get soft (yes, my microwave was working properly). Here is another method – more labour-intensive but it works.

1. Boil the halved potatoes for 6–7 minutes, drain and dry on kitchen paper.
2. Cut into thickish slices and brown either in the steak frying pan containing delicious meat residue (you will have to keep the meat warm without cooking it further in the meantime), or in another non-stick pan containing a teaspoon of olive oil, over a medium heat.
3. Stir the slices and turn them to ensure they are cooked through and evenly browned.

Strawberry Creams
Choose a sugarless jelly if you can find one.

1 strawberry jelly
$^{1}/_{2}$ litre ($^{3}/_{4}$ pint) boiling water
small can light evaporated milk

1.   Pull or cut the jelly into cubes, place in a bowl and pour over boiling water. It is quite capable of dissolving almost unaided, but you should give it a stir to start it off and after 5–10 minutes to get it completely into solution.
2.   When it has cooled slightly, stir in the milk. Pour into one large dish or individual glasses to set in fridge.

Day 7

LUNCH
A small green starter salad of baby spinach leaves and halved cherry tomatoes, dressed with balsamic vinegar mixed with any finely chopped fresh herbs.

Tiffany Eggs
This can be the main dish of a weekend brunch, or lunch any day when you have the time to prepare something luscious for yourself and Significant Other(s).

4 medium to large free-range eggs at room temperature
115g (4oz) smoked salmon, cut into slivers or
115g (4oz) tinned salmon, pink or red or
85–115g (3–4oz) fresh salmon, poached and flaked
freshly milled black pepper
2 tsp chives, very finely cut
light mayonnaise

1.   Place eggs in a small saucepan and just cover with cold water. Bring to the boil. Reduce to a simmer, and cook for exactly 3 minutes.
2.   Run cold water over the eggs until cool enough to handle, then gently crack open one end, discarding the 'hat'. Scrape the insides

(which should consist of firm but not rubbery white and gloriously runny yolk) into a small basin, setting shells aside.

3. Add the salmon, pepper and chives to the eggs and mix well, moistening with a little of the tinned or poaching liquid if using, or 1–2 tsp of a bland, light mayonnaise.

4. Pack mixture gently back into the shells, and serve with light rye or other bread of your choice, or make your own fresh Gypsy Melba Toast (see below).

Gypsy Melba Toast

White bread, it has to be said, works best for Melba Toast, but it's your choice.

1–2 medium-thick slices of bread per person
reduced-fat butter or soft margarine
a small, sharp knife
patience!

1. Toast each slice to a golden brown. Wait for a few seconds until cool enough to handle, then place slice flat on work surface. Holding firm with one hand, slip the knife blade into the uncooked 'middle', starting at one corner. Gently slide the blade along as though skinning a fish, until you have two slices in place of one.

2. For Melba Toast, brown the untoasted sides and eat at once, or allow to cool before storing in an air-tight tin.

3. For Gypsy Toast, just butter the untoasted side.

4. For Gypsy Melba, butter uncooked side then toast under grill.

Fresh mango or grapes.

DINNER
Slice of melon dressed with powdered cinnamon or ginger; or finely
chopped preserved ginger and a little of the syrup.
Roast lamb and mint sauce, potatoes, peas and carrots.

Apple Snow
680g (1$^1/_2$ lb) cooking apples (windfalls are fine for this), peeled, cored
and sliced
115ml (4fl oz/$^1/_2$ cup) water
an inch or so of lemon peel (no pith)
$^1/_2$ tsp coriander seeds, if liked
3–4 egg whites
3 dessertspoons sugar

1. Cook apples in water until soft, together with lemon peel and
    coriander seeds tied in a piece of muslin (5–7 minutes). Sieve or
    liquidize, and set aside.
2. Place egg whites in a clean, dry bowl, and whisk until they form
    firm peaks. Fold in the sugar and then the cool cooked apple a tbsp
    at a time until fully blended.
3. Chill and serve.

Chapter six

Helpful Dietary Supplements

For a long time controversies have raged, and they continue to rage, about the need for supplementing the diet with natural nutrients. Unexpectedly, the agonists and antagonists are not segregated exclusively on either side of the dividing line between orthodox medicine and natural therapies. Some nutritionally-trained medical experts support nutrient supplementation, and take the naturopathic view that even an exclusively whole food diet must frequently fail to supply every vitamin, mineral, trace element and amino acid that an individual requires.

A few alternative practitioners support so strongly the benefits of whole food eating that they discourage supplementation, and point those whom they advise in the direction of an increasingly assiduous search for a perfectly balanced eating regimen.

Doubtless, as is always the case, there are points of truth on both sides. Theoretically, a whole food diet, containing adequate daily amounts of fresh, organically grown fruit and vegetables, their freshly squeezed juices; seeds, nuts and pulses; free range poultry and eggs; and fresh fish from pure, uncontaminated river and sea water should supply every nutrient the human body requires.

Practically, though, such a diet is impossible to follow, simply because many of the foods are unavailable: concentrating one's imaginative faculties and intellectual powers almost entirely upon the wholesomeness of one's next meal can increase stress levels and produce neurotic obsessiveness, while the frustrated individual remains continually dogged in his or her attempts.

MALNUTRITION IN THE WEST

In addition to this problem, the Western lifestyle, though termed affluent, brings with it a unique type of malnutrition, even for those who attempt to eat healthily. Hidden salt, fat and sugar are present in many proprietary brands of packet and frozen convenience health foods, and which of us, considering the pace at which most of us live, does not rely at least to some extent upon ready-prepared meals?

Stress plays a major part in all our lives from babyhood through to old age: the rising rate of stress-related diseases such as heart attacks, strokes and high blood pressure, psychosomatic illnesses and neurotic and psychotic disorders bears witness to this. Animal and human research studies carried out in Europe, the United States, Russia and Japan have shown that stress factors can have severely damaging effects upon both mind and body.

Once thought of as causing no more than tension and emotional problems, stress has now been shown to affect the function of the neuro-transmitter brain chemicals carrying electrical impulse messages throughout the brain, the immune defence system, in particular the white lymphocyte cells responsible for combating infectious illnesses and malignant cell change, and the production of hormones, enzymes and other essential body chemicals. The sum total of the effects of stress greatly increases our need for many, if not all, vital nutrients.

Other disruptive factors – such as geopathic stress (magnetic earth meridians, ley lines, etc.); electromagnetic interference from overhead power cables, VDUs, microwaves, televisions and other domestic and industrial appliances; atmospheric pollutants; fatigue; tobacco smoke;

chemically synthesized food additives; high alcohol consumption; radiation; and viral illnesses – also take their toll and increase our need for dietary supplementation.

SUPPLEMENTS FOR HIGH BLOOD PRESSURE AND THE CIRCULATION

Whatever supplementation plan you follow, always start by taking one multi-vitamin/mineral complex daily. Specific dietary nutrients found to help reduce raised blood pressure, especially when taken in conjunction with a whole food diet and other health measures, include the following.

Vitam E with Selenium

Vitamin E has a number of beneficial effects throughout the body, particularly upon blood vessels. It acts as an anti-blood-clotting agent and as an antioxidant, counteracting the effects of free radicals (highly active molecule fragments) which injure and destroy many tissues throughout the body, and are thought to increase the rate at which fatty deposits of atheroma are laid down on the walls of arteries. This vitamin also promotes the production of normal red blood cells, and the healthy growth and development of every organ, including the heart and circulatory system.

Vitamin E combats hypertension by maintaining the health of the heart, arteries, veins and capillaries, and by encouraging the balancing control of the dilation and construction of the arterioles, largely responsible for the level of the diastolic blood pressure. Its actions in this capacity are reflected in its long established benefits to menopausal women suffering from hot flushes and night sweats. These symptoms, occurring under the influence of a falling oestrogen level, are believed to result from diminished control of the expansion and contraction of small blood vessels situated in and immediately below the skin. Vitamin E has no direct effect upon oestrogen deficiency, but acts as a regulator of abnormal blood vessel activity.

Vitamin E's actions in enhancing sexual and athletic performance, improving acne and combating infertility are probably also related to its actions upon blood vessel function.

Natural sources include apricot oil, almonds, corn oil, cottonseed oil, hazelnuts (filberts), margarine, peanuts, sunflower seeds, wheatgerm, walnuts and wholewheat flour.

How to take: doses of 100 IU daily, building up to a dose of 400 IU daily, over a period of eight weeks, have been used successfully to treat hypertension. Consult your doctor or a qualified nutritional expert if you are receiving medication of any kind.

Vitamin E supplements are often found in combination with the trace element selenium. Trace elements are vital minerals required by the body in minute amounts. Selenium complements vitamin E as an antioxidant, functions as an antioxidant itself, and also promotes normal growth and development. It is also speculated to offer protection against all ageing mechanisms, which must include the clogging of arteries with atheromatous deposits; and it helps to counteract cardiovascular disease, heart attacks and strokes. It stimulates the immune defence system's cells, which also help to combat atheroma; it decreases platelet clumping in the bloodstream, and helps to prevent clot formation at the site of blood vessel damage in the heart and brain.

It occurs naturally in the following foods: wheatgerm and whole grain products, fish, liver and kidney, chicken, egg yolk, bran, broccoli, milk, mushrooms, cucumbers, garlic, cabbage and onions.

How to take: No UK RDA (Recommended Daily Amount) has been established, but the quantities found in combination with vitamin E supplements have been calculated to supply normal daily requirements.

Carnitine

Carnitine is one of about 20 amino acid building blocks from which protein is made. Like other members of this group of compounds, it plays several important biochemical roles in human and animal biochemistry. The most important of these, in the present context, is the transportation of fatty acids into the power houses (*mitochondria*), within which fatty acids and glucose combine with oxygen to produce energy.

According to recent research, carnitine appears to offer considerable benefit to the heart muscle of people suffering from atheromatous coronary arteries. Heart muscle cells are naturally rich in carnitine, one reason being that heart muscle derives between 48 and 70 per cent of its total energy requirements from long chain fatty acids. These energy requirements, even at rest, are considerable, for, unlike other bodily muscles, it can never take time off to relax. Over a 24-hour period, it pumps the equivalent of 1,800 gallons of blood through around 75,000 miles of blood vessels throughout the body.

High blood pressure strains the heart muscle, increasing its workload and its energy requirements. In a recent clinical study, intravenous carnitine was administered to patients with ischaemic (coronary) heart disease. Their exercise tolerance improved, and their heart muscles were discovered to make more efficient use of fatty acids as energy fuel.

Carnitine can be taken as a dietary supplement for its protective effect against cardiovascular disease, and to help strengthen weakened heart muscle. A suitable dose for most adults, with the former aim in view, is 200 mg three times daily. Individuals suffering from heart disease or high blood pressure should obtain medical advice from a nutritionally-oriented medical practitioner.

Other Amino Acids

Histidine improves the flow of blood in the coronary arteries, and helps to lower an elevated blood pressure by relaxing blood vessel walls.

Taurine has been used successfully as a treatment for congestive heart failure, a common complication of longstanding hypertension, as explained earlier (*see pages 37–38*). Over a four-week period, 58 sufferers took part in a controlled medical trial. Half of them received 'dummy' placebo tablets, while the rest received 6 grams of taurine daily. Those in the latter group experienced considerable relief from breathlessness, swelling and palpitations, while other benefits were noted in their chest X-ray pictures and in their overall functional capacity. Taurine proved useful whether or not the patients were received digitalis heart drugs. No significant improvement occurred in patients who received the 'dummies'.

In addition, taurine helps to keep cholesterol in solution in the bloodstream, rather than solidifying into plaques within arterial walls.

Fish Oil Supplements

These are known to contain *essential fatty acids* offering considerable and effective protection against heart and arterial disease. The most important is EPA (eicosapentaenoic acid), a continually high intake of which has been causally related to the low incidence of coronary thrombosis and other forms of heart disease in Greenland Eskimos, Japanese fishing communities and other populations with a high consumption of oily fish.

EPA gives rise to compounds known as 3-series PGs, a class of prostaglandins, or hormone-like substances, which play vital roles in the minute-by-minute regulation of cellular processes throughout the body. The 3-series PG make blood clot formation (thrombosis) less likely, so EPA not only reduces the risk of heart attacks and strokes, but also lowers the levels of the class of blood fats and cholesterol most likely to give rise to fatty arterial plaques. It has also been shown to lower blood pressure, and to affect the activity of the monocytes (a class of white blood cell) which help to combat arterial disease throughout the body.

EPA may also help to reduce high blood pressure. One clinical trial involved 16 hypertensive patients over a 12-week period. All participants had a systolic blood pressure below 200 mm Hg, and a diastolic blood pressure between 91–100 mm Hg.

They were randomly allotted to one or other of two groups; all received a 'dummy' placebo oil and a pure fish oil supplement in turn. The study was 'double-blind', i.e. neither doctors nor patients knew until the trial was over which patients had received olive oil placebo and which fish oil at any given moment during the study.

The average blood pressure of the patients, before they were allotted to their two groups, was 160/94 mm Hg. Following six weeks on placebo oil, this average had risen to 161/94.5 mm Hg; and after fish oil supplementation it had dropped to 151/92.5 mm Hg. In a reclining position, the systolic blood pressure was lower after fish oil extract than after olive oil placebo by an average of 5.48 per cent; and in a vertical position, i.e. standing, by an average of 5.66 per cent. The reduction in diastolic blood pressure following fish oil extract was not statistically significant.

Of the 16 patients, 13 found fish oil extract either as acceptable as, or more acceptance than, previous medication they had received for hypertension. The fish oil supplement used in this trial contained a higher concentration of EPA than those available in chemists and health food shops for a purely protective purpose; nevertheless, taking a daily fish oil supplement is a wise and healthy practice, whether your aim is to improve your overall health, vitality and cardiac stamina, or counteract high blood pressure naturally.

Evening Primrose Oil

Evening primrose oil contains the essential fatty acid GLA (Gamma-linolenic acid) which also gives rise to helpful, heart-protective prostaglandins, this time of the 1-series (PGE1s). Efamol is the brand that has been used in numerous clinical trials and studies evaluating the wide range of GLA's therapeutic applications, which have shown between 4 and 8 500 mg captules of Efamol, taken daily, lower blood cholesterol levels, reduce the risks of thrombosis and can be highly effective in lowering blood pressure in patients suffering from mild to moderate hypertension.

Coenzyme Q

This nutrient has attracted much research interest over the past decade. Coenzyme Q (CoQ) is an essential constituent of the cells' mitochondria, and it plays a vital role in energy production. Oxygen plays an essential part in the energy equation, and, as we have seen, unites with glucose and long chain essential fatty acids within heart muscular tissue, to release necessary energy. Specifically, it controls the flow of oxygen within individual cells, and therefore plays a major role in the metabolism of heart muscle.

Tests have shown that CoQ can lower blood pressure, relieve angina and counteract congestive heart failure by enhancing the heart's muscular activity. Consult your doctor or a medically-qualified nutritionist before taking this nutrient, if you suffer from heart disease or other circulatory problems.

ANTI-STRESS SUPPLEMENTS

Vitamin C with Bioflavonoids

Vitamin C is the anti-stress vitamin par excellence. It boosts the immune defence system against the effects of physical, mental and emotional strain, and aids iron absorption essential to the production of haemoglobin, the oxygen carrying blood pigment, and of healthy red cells in the bone marrow.

It keeps the capillaries strong and healthy, and helps to guard against the weakness of their walls, leading to the leaking of blood following a bruise injury. Present in high concentration in citrus fruits, vitamin C was first discovered when oranges, lemons and limes were found to cure scurvy, the main symptoms of which are heavy bruising following minor injuries, and bleeding gums.

Other benefits of vitamin C supplementation include a reduction in blood cholesterol level, protection against heart disease and improvement in emotional, stress-related disorders.

Natural sources of Vitamin C, besides citrus fruits, include: spinach, cabbage, broccoli, Brussels sprouts, watercress, green peppers (capsicum), kale, tomatoes, potatoes, paw-paws (papaya), guavas, rosehips and black-currants.

How to take: Opinion varies enormously about the amount of vitamin C we should take as a daily supplement. Doctor Linus Pauling, the famous pioneer research scientist and Nobel prize winner, is reputed to have cured cancer with very high doses of intravenous vitamin C, and to take in the region of 21 grams daily himself. Generally, one gram daily, in addition to the vitamin C present in your multi-vitamin/mineral complex, should suffice; you should be able, safely, to double or treble this dose for a few days when symptoms of a cold, sore throat or influenza appear, or when under heavy strain.

Bioflavonoids are the brightly coloured pigments in the skin and flesh of citrus fruits, peppers, apricots, cherries, grapes, paw-paws, tomatoes and in green leafy vegetables. They are found in association with vitamin C, and include rutin, hesperidin, nobiletin, sinensetin and tangeretin.

They, too, have an antioxidant effect, preventing the oxidation of vitamin C and adrenaline by copper-containing enzymes. They strengthen capillaries; prevent nosebleeds, post-partum (after birth) haemorrhage and easy bruising. They may also help to counteract retinal bleeding at the back of the eye in people with diabetes and hypertension.

How to take: No RDA has yet been established, but the amount present in vitamin C supplements is sufficient for normal purposes. Do not take it to rectify a bleeding problem without consulting your doctor first about the underlying cause.

Vitamin B Complex

A need for B-complex vitamins increases generally when we are under stress. Supplementation with certain of them is known to offer particular value; unless advised differently by a qualified nutritionist, you should take the entire complex in one supplement. Thiamine (vitamin B$_1$) helps to combat emotional highs and lows. Niacin (vitamin B$_3$) promotes the health of the entire nervous system, and helps to protect against both migraine headaches and stress-related high blood pressure. Pantothenic acid (vitamin B$_5$) relieves tension, aids adrenal gland function and combats anxiety and fatigue caused by subjection to physical/psychological stress. Pyridoxine (vitamin B$_6$) can offer effective relief from tension and anxiety caused by the premenstrual syndrome (PMS).

Calcium

Many nutritional experts, doctors and natural therapists recommend calcium supplements when stress levels are high, in order to meet the body's extra demands for calcium. Smokers and high protein eaters share an increased need for this mineral. Before, during and after the menopause, women are particularly in need of calcium, since a falling oestrogen level encourages bone thinning (osteoporosis). The menopause, which generally occurs in the West around the age of 50, is also the age at which weight problems, cardiovascular disease and hypertension are most likely to become apparent. The menopause itself also gives rise to additional tension, stress, worry and irritability.

Calcium supplements taken before retiring can help to ensure a sound night's sleep.

Magnesium

This has been dubbed the anti-stress mineral. It is essential for calcium and vitamin C metabolism, and should be taken with calcium in half the former mineral's dose.

The majority of people under stress require extra magnesium, while heavy drinkers need even more. Besides combating depression and tension, magnesium promotes the health of the cardiovascular system and helps to prevent heart attacks. (See *The Vitamin Bible*, Earl Mindell, Arlington Books 1985).

Zinc

This mineral plays many essential roles in the body. It combats tension, helps to maintain mental alertness, and counteracts certain types of depression.

Chapter seven

Easy Exercise

Many people – especially those of us who could best make use of it – remain unconvinced of the value of regular physical exercise. The prospect of becoming more active can seem depressing and daunting, especially when we already feel overtired at the end of a busy day in the home or at work.

Driving in congested cities, travelling on public transport, shopping, housework and looking after small children, often in addition to hours spent in an office, factory or other place of employment, can make us too exhausted even to learn to relax! So it is little wonder that exercise is generally at the bottom of the list of health measures we are prepared to introduce into our daily lifestyle.

Nevertheless, exercise is proving a key factor in the treatment of both hypertension and cardiovascular disease. Monitored exercise is the key to the high success rate of the Cardiovascular Rehabilitation Centre at Houston, Texas. During its first seven years (1978–85), the Centre treated more than 1,000 patients, all of whom had been seriously ill, and about half of whom began treatment at risk of sudden death at any moment.

According to a report by David Loshat in *GP* (21st June 1985), 10 out of 12 patients who were waiting for heart transplant operations regained sufficiently good health to permit them to return to work and a normal life. The Centre's director and founder, Dr Lysle Peterson, former President of the International Cardiological Society, found that all the patients treated had improved their heart condition by 300 per cent, regardless of their age. In addition, their use of diuretic, vasodilator and beta blocker drugs had fallen by an overall 63 per cent.

All treatment was carried out at the Centre on a day-patient basis, and a rehabilitation course lasted for around 14 weeks, comprising two hours a day three times weekly.

Not only is this form of treatment far more cost-effective, but it also achieves better effects than surgery and medication, although these still play a part in the management of a number of individuals.

The Centre used a stationary exercise bicycle, since this provides a simple method of providing precisely the amount of exercise a patient needs, and for monitoring his or her heart beat and blood pressure. While jogging, squash, etc. can be dangerous for heart patients, stationary cycling at a predetermined therapeutic level had never resulted in the need to resuscitate a single patient, despite some of them being over 88 years old.

A more recent study in the US was supported by the National Heart, Lung and Blood Institute (reported in *Journal of the American Medical Association*, 27 January 1999). 'Project Active' enrolled 235 men and women, aged between 35 and 60. At the time of enrolment, all were free of heart and arterial disease but had sedentary lifestyles and were moderately overweight. Of these volunteers, 122 were assigned to a lifestyle management group (A) where they learned behavioural skills to increase their daily physical activity, while 113 were assigned to the more structured group (B) where they used a fitness centre for traditional vigorous exercise such as aerobics, stair-climbing and swimming. Both groups learned behavioural skills to increase activity, but group A members received more individual help in restructuring their lifestyle. The researchers found that, after six months, group B had attained better heart and lung fitness than group A, but this declined rapidly once vigorous exercise ceased. After two years, however, both groups had significantly improved heart and lung function and clinically significant lower blood pressure. Most participants maintained this BP and cardiorespiratory improvement long term. Small changes in lifestyle to increase physical activity are therefore as beneficial as systematic aerobic training.

THE EFFECTS OF EXERCISE

Healthy exercise training works on the overload principle. That is, you need to make only a little greater effort when performing it than that to which you are already accustomed. Two swimming-bath lengths of the crawl stroke may be sufficient for you in the early stages if you are unfit, whereas 40–50 lengths may be needed at a faster pace for a competitive swimmer. If you are not used to walking for many minutes at a time, 20–30 minutes spent walking briskly at around 3 mph will produce beneficial physiological and biochemical changes.

These include extra oxygen being extracted by the muscles of the body from the blood, and a reduced demand upon the heart muscle. Your resting heart rate becomes lower, and, when exercising, you will find your heart beating less rapidly than before, although it retains the full strength of its beat and output of blood. The muscles become more adept at extracting available oxygen, so less oxygenated arterial blood is required to reach them. This means that when you really have to exert yourself unexpectedly, the effects upon your physiological processes and cardiovascular system will be far less drastic. In addition, once the heart starts to contract more effectively at each beat, and the rate at which it beats is reduced, the heart's muscle is spared much unnecessary work. These mechanisms help to explain the beneficial effects of exercise on the heart and blood vessels, and on other bodily systems.

BENEFITS OF EXERCISE

In an article which appeared in *The Practitioner* (December 1987, Vol. 231), entitled 'Reasons for Advising Exercise', the authors, Joan Bassey, Peter Fentem and Nancy Turnbull of the Department of Physiology and Pharmacology, Queens Medical Centre, Nottingham, underline the advantages of regular exercise under several headings. Significantly, regular, increased physical activity seems to inhibit the rise in blood pressure, and reduce the frequency of arterial hypertension in previously healthy men and women as they grow older.

They say:

> In several intervention studies, adults with mild/moderate or labile systematic arterial hypertension ... showed an average reduction of 13/10 millimetres Hg in arterial blood pressure with regular, moderate, endurance exercise. Hypertensive adolescents, and severely hypertensive women also showed reductions. This reduction in blood pressure may represent one mechanism by which physical activity contributes to the prevention of coronary heart disease and stroke.

Coronary Heart Disease

There is a proven direct relationship between regular physical exercise and a healthy heart. Exercise that makes a demand upon the heart (aerobic exercise) increases its strength in the ways described above, and reduces the major known risk factors to coronary heart disease. Besides reducing blood pressure, it lowers the blood fat level, discourages clot formation (thrombosis), helps maintain a normal body weight and releases emotional tension.

The importance of the last-mentioned factor is reflected in the 'Type A' personality profile which has been shown to be associated with a higher than normal risk of suffering a heart attack. Type A people tend to react badly to stress, become tense and frequently irritable, and characteristically worry about trivia; they also tend to be perfectionists, and 'high achievers'. Regular exercise is of particular benefit to people of this type since it offers an opportunity for a release of their pent-up energy and tension.

While regular, monitored exercise cannot replace damaged heart tissue with new, living cells following a coronary thrombosis, its overall benefits are felt by the rest of the healthy heart muscle. Recovery after a heart attack, when exercise is used as part of the treatment regimen, is normally more rapid and more successful, and the resultant feeling of getting back to 'normal' helps to relieve the melancholic forebodings from which many heart attack patients suffer.

Claudication

Doctors also recommend daily regular exercise for the treatment of arterial problems in other body areas. Diseased arteries in the legs cause cramping pain and a limp (claudication) when walking, because the leg muscles' extra demand for oxygen and nutrients is failing to be met by the diminished blood supply. While arterial surgery can 'declog' and sometimes replace sections of diseased peripheral arteries, many physicians and vascular surgeons now prefer the more conservative approach of a carefully controlled, gradually-increasing walking regimen. Regular leg exercise of this type, carried out by many scores of patients, has proved highly beneficial, since it has been found to result in the growth of new blood vessels in the affected leg muscles. This results in patients being able to walk further, without claudication symptoms, over a period of weeks or months.

Osteoporosis

Exercise also helps to combat the bone-thinning disease, osteoporosis. All adults lose calcium from their bones from around the age of 35 onwards, but the condition is particularly serious in women, who lose considerably more than men in their late 40s and early 50s when the menopause takes place and their blood oestrogen levels fall. Osteoporotic bones become brittle and fracture easily. The most serious fracture affecting elderly women is that of the neck of the femur (the upper end of the long thigh bone as it enters the hip joint): 15 per cent of patients with this injury die within three months, and the condition costs the National Health Service in excess of £100 million annually.

Diabetes

Diabetics run an increased risk of developing diseased, fat-clogged arteries and other vascular problems. Exercise proves useful in this capacity since it improves tolerance to carbohydrates and increases the body cells' sensitivity to whatever insulin the pancreas is able to produce.

Insomnia

A further bonus of exercise is the promotion of sound, healthy sleep. The demands of a busy, stressful lifestyle make adequate rest imperative, yet many exhausted individuals lie awake night after night, tossing, turning and fretting about daily worries which inevitably become magnified out of all proportion in the dark, small hours. Chronic insomnia can have an adverse effect on many aspects of health, and can put the thought of daily physical exertion out of the question.

Paradoxically, aerobic or 'demand' exercise tires you healthily; following it, tense, taut muscles relax, and a regular sleep pattern can often be re-established without the use of drugs.

Table 2: The effect of exercise on heart disease high risk factors

Blood pressure		
Systolic	↓	13 mm HG
Diastolic	↓	10 mm HG
Blood fat levels		
(lipoproteins)		
Healthy lipoproteins	↑	
Harmful lipoproteins	↓	
Total cholesterol	↓	
Triglycerides	↓	
Clotting factors		
Anticlotting function	↑	
Proclotting function	↓	(After vigorous exercise)
Metabolism		
Energy balance regulation	↑	
Heart		
Heart muscle work	↓	
Risk of irregular rhythms	↓	
Heart rate	↓	

HOW TO START

The best approach is to aim at taking regular exercise; for example, three 20–30 minute exercise sessions every week. The worst approach is to take up a very demanding sport such as squash, spend out on new clothes and equipment, and rush at your new project with unbridled enthusiasm when you haven't exercised for years. At best, you are likely to become rapidly exhausted and disillusioned, and give up exercising as quickly as you started, perhaps suffering a tendon, joint or soft tissue injury into the bargain. You may do yourself serious harm, and at worst, if you're very unfit and suffering from high blood pressure, may even bring on the heart attack you are seeking to avert.

Your choice of exercise should be based on two considerations. Most importantly, it should be a form of activity which you are likely to enjoy. Secondly, it should involve rhythmic action which makes use of the body's large muscle groups. Brisk walking and swimming are ideal. If you cannot swim, now is the time to learn. You may claim to dislike walking, and it is often an unpleasant experience when confined to hard pavements and busy, polluted streets. However, most urban areas are close to a park, common or open space, so buy some comfortable, good quality trainers, don a tracksuit or other loose comfortable clothing, and set out to become regularly acquainted with your local sample of the countryside.

The secret is to start modestly, and a further helpful hint is to avoid telling all and sundry of your new exercise scheme. Even well-meaning people frequently ridicule the health measures which they are not prepared to follow themselves, and sensing safety in numbers, they feel ill at ease until you relinquish your aims and rejoin their ranks.

Ask your doctor to check your heart and blood pressure first, before taking up exercise, if these have ever presented problems. Set yourself small goals initially, starting with 5–10 minutes of gentle exercise, and building up in gradual stages until you are well able to tolerate a full half hour of aerobic activity.

Do not confine exercise to your thrice-weekly training sessions. Start living more actively right away by climbing stairs instead of taking the lift, gradually increasing the storeys you walk up in a tall building. Take additional short walks wherever possible – if you normally get the car out to take a short trip to the newsagents or local shops, try leaving it behind! Join in with your children's or grandchildren's sports and games. Hopefully they'll be delighted at your participation, and you, and they, may learn a lot!

Always limber up for five minutes before and after an exercise session. Rotate your shoulder joints, gently flex your arm, wrist, hip, knee and ankle joints, and shake your arms about, loosening up your fingers.

Try to touch your toes – and don't be dismayed if this is impossible. One of the benefits of your exercise regimen will soon show itself to be improved joint and muscle flexibility.

Table 3: Exercising pulse rates by age and fitness

Age	Max heart rate	Exercise pulse rate (unfit)	Exercise pulse rate (fit)
16	204	123	164
18	202	122	162
20	200	120	160
22	198	119	158
24	196	118	157
26	194	116	155
28	192	115	154
30	190	114	152
32	188	113	150
34	186	112	149
36	184	110	147
38	182	109	146
40	180	108	144
45	175	105	140
50	170	102	136
55	165	99	132
60	160	96	128
65	155	93	124
70	150	90	120
75	145	87	116
80	140	84	112

Finally, run slowly and gently on the spot. Table 3 shows the pulse rates at which to aim when exercising, according to your age and fitness. Refer to the higher of two ages, if you are between them. *Do not aim* to reach your maximum heart rate (second column). This figure is used to calculate the level to which your pulse should rise for you to benefit, and is calculated by subtracting your age in years from 220. Your pulse rate should reach 60 per cent of the maximum heart rate if you are unfit, and 80 per cent if you are fit.

As you will see, the age column extends from 16 to 80 years. According to a report in *Geriatric Medicine* (May 1986), only a proportion of decline in elderly people results from the disease process; much of it is caused by underuse. For a variety of reasons, including stiffness, pain and weakness, elderly people make less use of a particular part of their body and become less active, in this way widening the gap between possible and actual fitness. Oxford Community Physician, J. A. Muir Gray, pointed out in the report that many veterans' sporting records demonstrate that the loss of fitness due to age alone is a great deal less than most people, including many doctors, would imagine.

'There is every reason to encourage people to try to keep fit as they grow older as a way of preventing some of the problems typical of old age,' said Dr Muir Gray. He referred to encouraging evidence which suggests that fitness can be regained in old age: in one study, seven weeks' conditioning improved oxygen-demanding power activity by 30 per cent, and 'maximum oxygen intake was brought quite quickly to the level anticipated in a sedentary person ten to twenty years younger than the test subject'. Other research studies suggest that suppleness, strength and skill, in addition to stamina, can be significantly improved in elderly people.

The following table appeared in *Geriatric Medicine* (May 1986):

Table 4: Fit veterans' peak performance is surprisingly close to that of their younger counterparts (British Veterans' cycling records, 1983)

25 miles		50 miles		100 miles	
Age	Time	Age	Time	Age	Time
43	52.45	43	1.47.38	43	3.51.25
66	57.05	66	2.52.41	66	4.16.37
77	1.08.00	77	2.19.57	76	5.16.53
82	1.37.00	78	2.52.38		

Relaxation Techniques

As we saw during the earlier discussion upon the effects of stress, prolonged tension and worry, combined with adverse factors in our social and/or domestic environment, increase the release of the stress hormones adrenaline and nora-drenaline into the bloodstream. This process is in fact just one highly important aspect of a wide spectrum of neurophysiological processes triggered by stress, and resulting from stimulation of the autonomic nervous system.

As its name applies, the autonomic nervous system functions outside our conscious control. It regulates bodily functions such as our heartbeat, respiration, hormone release and the multitude of physiological and bio-chemical processes which continue to function independently of any effort that we can make, day and night, throughout our entire lives.

This part of our nervous system functions by reflex action. The majority of bodily functions are controlled in this way, including the dila-tion and constriction of blood vessels in the skin in response to external temperature change, the constriction of the pupils of the eye to bright light, and the production of saliva immediately before, and during, eating.

The autonomic nervous system comprises two discrete sets of nerves. Many organs, blood vessels and glands receive nerve fibres from both, their function being regulated by the balance of their opposed activity.

Sympathetic nerves arise from small collections of nerve cells called ganglia, found in pairs throughout the greater part of the spinal cord. Messages from the brain to the sympathetic ganglia generate impulses in sympathetic nerve fibres, generally resulting in the release of adrenaline and noradrenaline in the parts of the body and tissues that they supply.

While the function of the sympathetic nervous system is closely related to blood pressure increase, its counterpart, the parasympathetic nervous system, has the reverse effect. Parasympathetic nerves arise in the body in two main groups. The most important of these, the vagus nerve, arises from the base of the brain, travels down among the structures of the neck to the thorax (chest) where it sends off branches to the heart, and travels downwards through the diaphragm into the abdomen where it sends vital branches to the stomach, increasing, among other factors, the secretion of hydrochloric acid during the process of digestion.

The second portion of the parasympathetic nervous system arises from the lower end of the spinal cord, and is intimately connected with the function of the bladder and other pelvic organs. In contrast to the sympathetic nervous system, the parasympathetic functions by releasing the neurotransmitter chemical messenger, acetylcholine, from its terminal nerve endings.

Besides transferring messages from the brain and central nervous system, the autonomic nerves also relay sensation from the bodily organs to the brain. In some instances, these result in reflex effects in appropriate bodily areas, and do not reach our conscious awareness. A rise in blood pressure, for instance, reaches the brain and results in nerve stimuli travelling by the vagus parasympathetic nerves to the heart muscle, to decrease its activity. The fact that many high blood pressure sufferers have a fast pulse rate in addition to hypertension reflects the fact that their sympathetic nerves are currently in 'overdrive', i.e. they are overriding the beneficial effects of the parasympathetic nerves. Certain autonomic nervous system messages *do* reach conscious awareness. A sudden shock, accident or unpleasant sight can send alarm messages racing through our autonomic nervous system, which result in immediate nausea and vomiting. In this case, awareness of sympathetic/parasympathetic activity is both strong and unpleasant.

HARNESSING PARASYMPATHETIC POWER

Many modern psychologically orientated therapies, especially those stemming from the United States, have over the past two decades urged us to get into contact with our 'inner selves' by a variety of means. While increased insight into our mental make-up and the way our bodies function is largely to be applauded, some proponents of 'getting in touch' techniques go overboard in their enthusiasm. The suggestions made in this book for getting in touch with your parasympathetic nervous system are urbane and, above all, practicable.

Parasympathetic activity counteracts the sympathetic nervous system processes that are largely responsible for generating high blood pressure. While sympathetic activity can best be visualized by imagining yourself in a 'flight or fight' situation, with tense muscles, dilated pupils, a rapid heart beat, quick shallow breathing and some of your hairs literally standing on end, parasympathetic activity can best be understood by imagining yourself asleep in an armchair after a large lunch.

In this instance, your body's main need is to divert extra blood to your stomach and bowel, to aid the process of digestion. The muscles of your arms, legs, and trunk are loose and relaxed; your eyelids are closed, your pupils constricted, your heartbeat normal to slow, and your breathing even, deep and regular. Moreover, instead of large quantities of adrenaline and noradrenaline pouring into your blood stream from your adrenal glands, your body's main hormonal concern is directed towards the release of digestive enzymes in response to your meal. Most important, in the present context, your blood pressure is normal or as low as it is likely to get if you already suffer from hypertension.

Doctors and other health experts have coined the term trophotropic to describe the response of the parasympathetic nervous system. Its activities are those of slowing, tranquillizing and inhibiting sympathetic activity, and restoring both mind and body to a state of balance and harmony. Relaxation techniques produce this condition, and are increasingly used by both doctors and alternative practitioners since deep relaxation has been found highly conducive to positive health. Conditions known to benefit include tachycardia (a fast heart beat), palpitations and high blood pressure, together with a wide spectrum of anxiety symptoms, so often found in association with hypertension. These include sleep problems, irritability and tension, fatigue, exhaustion and reactive depression. Other related symptoms comprise hyperventilation (rapid breathing), nausea, shakiness, panic attacks, phobias, dizziness, migraine, asthma and premenstrual syndrome (PMS).

In her feature 'The Use of Relaxation Techniques in General Practice', Julienne McLean M.Sc., Medical Psychologist at the Department of General Practice, St Mary's Hospital Medical School, London, discusses neuromuscular relaxation and meditation in the treatment of high blood pressure and other conditions, as described below.

Neuromuscular Relaxation

This relaxation method reduces tension and nerve activity in the muscles of the body under our conscious control. Progressive muscular relaxation, developed by Edmund Jacobson, is a popular form. Jacobson emphasizes the value of the individual learning the difference between tension and relaxation, and his method consists of the contraction, followed by the relaxation, of selected muscles and muscle groups throughout the body. A state of deep relaxation follows the treatment of all the main body muscles in this manner. Some therapists advocate contracting and relaxing several muscle groups at a time, e.g. the left leg, arm and side of the abdomen, while others favour working up the body from feet to skull, contracting smaller muscle groups in a more systematic way. Thus, the subject may be instructed first to contract and relax the muscles of the left foot, noting the sensations, and to follow this by repeating the exercise with the right foot.

Some practitioners prefer to use a passive rather than a physically active form of relaxation. The basis of this variation is getting the patient to focus his or her attention on a series of individual muscle groups, and then relaxing them through a process of direct concentration. Here, the use of mental imagery is important, the patient being asked to visualize, for example, and then feel – i.e. be aware of – the muscles of the left calf, thigh, abdomen etc.

It has been suggested that anxiety can be split into thought-orientated and body-orientated forms, localized in the two hemispheres of the brain, and that different forms of relaxation are appropriate for different types of anxiety. Two researchers, Davidson and Schwartz (1976), who have delved deeply into the subject, have suggested that progressive muscular relaxation is the most effective form of treatment for body-orientated anxiety. It has been found highly effective in the treatment of essential hypertension, sleep problems, migraine, tension headaches and other aspects of anxiety, including psychosomatic pain. Sometimes, other forms of treatment for a patient's stress need to include behaviour therapy or other forms of psychotherapy as adjuncts to relaxation.

Meditation

In her discussion of this subject, Julienne McLean points out that although it has been used for thousands of years 'within the religious and philosophical traditions of the east', only for the past 30 years has it been used as a form of medical and psychotherapeutic treatment without religious connotations. All meditation techniques make use of a focal device, upon which the individual concentrates his or her attention. This may be a visual image, such as a mandala, or a flower; physical activity such as dancing, breathing or jogging; or mental repetition, such as a mantra, prayer or chant. Euphonious, flowing words should be chosen with care for their suitability to the individual patient, and phrases involving several words should have a positive, confidence-boosting meaning.

Meditation brings about the trophotropic state by encouraging the intuitive type of thought pattern characteristic of the brain's right hemisphere to predominate in the individual's consciousness rather than the usually dominant, analytical thought mode progressing from the left hemisphere. Physiological changes reported to take place during meditation include slowing of the heart rate, a reduced oxygen consumption, decreased respiration rate, an increased regularity of alpha brain wave activity and a reduction in blood pressure. These responses are not unique to meditation, it is now believed, but common to all passive relaxation techniques. Research studies into the use of meditation in reducing high blood pressure have consistently shown a reduction in blood pressure in the treatment group, a reduction in the use of antihypertensive drugs, and a reduction in bodily symptoms. Follow-up data have shown that treatment gains were maintained over a 12-month period and also after four years.

Biofeedback Training

Biofeedback training is a method of monitoring bodily functions, and using information gained about them to bring about necessary and desirable changes. Our bodies utilize the principle of feedback in order to operate as an integral whole. The sympathetic nervous system uses it when we are subjected to stress. Emotions such as fear or excitement, arising in the cortex of the brain, send stimuli to the hypothalamus in the mid-brain, which in turn helps to generate impulses in the sympathetic nervous system. In this example of biofeedback, data from the brain's emotional centres is 'fed' to the hypothalamus, which utilizes it to set in motion the necessary sympathetic response.

Biofeedback calls into action a function of the human mind that has been explored most fully in the past by the use of hypnotism. Hypnosis has been used experimentally to cause a number of bodily changes such as an increase in skin temperature, and the disappearance of rashes, warts, etc. It works by harnessing the power of the subconscious mind while the individual is in a hypnotic trance. Biofeedback is now used to give people a high degree of control over physiological events that were once thought to be outside conscious control. Biofeedback training seems to make non-sense of the statement made earlier in this chapter that the autonomic nervous system governs those bodily functions outside the control of the conscious mind. The contradiction is only a partial one, however.

Biofeedback training has been used in Western medicine for around 30 years, and hundreds of papers have been written about its use. In prac-tical terms, it is carried out by a doctor or therapist by attaching the patient to some kind of electronic or electrical apparatus, which monitors a particular output from a bodily system, and displays the results in such a way, visibly or audibly, that the person can keep a constant tab on the suc-cess of his efforts. If, for example, he is asked to 'try to relax', successful achievement of this task may be reflected by a loud hum, or a row of coloured lights. It is difficult to tell a person how to relax, so biofeedback training marshals a person's innate awareness of how this is done. It is very difficult indeed to try to explain, for example, how to ride a bicycle. This can only be learned by the method of trial and error, and involves practis-ing to the point at which you 'get the feel' of the degree of balance and muscular co-ordination required. One method uses a galvanic skin response (GSR) device which picks up tiny quantities of perspiration on the skin of the subject's fingertips. The greater the state of tension, the greater the perspiration output. As the tension is replaced by a more relaxed state, less perspiration is produced, thereby acquainting the person with what has to be done in order to achieve tranquility of mind and body.

In an instance such as this, no complicated instructions are given. Subjects undergoing the training usually start by relaxing their bodily muscles, only to discover that success is partial, i.e. the machine is produc-ing a hum at half its normal pitch, or only some of the coloured lights on the machine have lit up. They then generally try out the effects of different frames of mind. This could include visualizing a restful scene such as a beach or a woodland glade, or imagining oneself surrounded by a bubble of clear blue light. What works for one individual is usually peculiar to him or her, and may not be effective for another subject.

Excellent results have been obtained using biofeedback training in combination with yoga, meditation and other specific relaxation techniques. Doctors Chandra Patel and W.R.S. North reported the results of a study in *The Lancet* (19 July 1975). Working with 34 patients suffering from high blood pressure, they organized two forms of treatment to which the patients were randomly assigned – one was a 'placebo' therapy consisting of general relaxation, and the other was a combination of yoga relaxation methods and biofeedback training.

Both groups showed a reduction in blood pressure after the six week period. The average reading of the general relaxation group was reduced from 169/101 to 160/96 mm Hg, while the biofeedback/yoga group showed an average reduction from 168/100 to 141/84 mm Hg. Statistically, a fall of 16 mm Hg in diastolic blood pressure is extremely significant.

Doctors North and Patel used Jacobson's progressive relaxation techniques, discussed above, in the first instance, and then taught the relevant patients transcendental meditation. To increase the success of both methods, each patient involved was connected to two biofeedback machines giving a continuous audio signal whose pitch fell as relaxation was achieved. The first machine was a GSR device, and the second was a machine which measured electrical activity in muscles.

The doctors said in their report:

Patients were also encouraged verbally and were shown their blood pressure records; they were also instructed to practise relaxation and meditation twice a day, and gradually to try to incorporate these habits into routine activities, the methods depending upon individual circumstances. For example, each patient had a red disc attached to his watch to remind him to relax whenever he looked at the time, and some were told to relax before answering the telephone.

Many doctors feel that biofeedback equipment should be used only under professional supervision. Training devices are offered for sale to the public, and most intelligent people can use such a machine successfully in order to teach themselves how to relax. However, it is most important to get medical advice before undertaking biofeedback training as a form of treatment.

Chapter nine

Cigarettes, Alcohol and Hypertension

Many would-be non-smokers believe that there is a secret which, if they learned it, would enable them to quit their habit successfully. This is true, and the secret is so simple that most people overlook it. It is no more, and no less, than actually *wanting* to quit the habit badly enough to make the effort.

The majority of smokers give up at some point in their lives – and some do so many times over. But frequently, the withdrawal symptoms from nicotine, and the loss of a long-established and familiar habit, cause them to restart. Smokers who do give up permanently achieve their goals just because they are determined to do so at all costs. If you have tried and failed, facing the facts about cigarettes, high blood pressure and premature death should help to give you the necessary willpower.

CIGARETTES AND YOUR BODY

All cigarette packets bear a warning along the lines that their contents can cause lung cancer, bronchitis and other chest diseases. If packets of biscuits or sweets bearing a similar message were introduced into the shops, there would be a public outcry. As it is, sales of cigarettes, tobacco and cigars continue.

Everyone knows that cigarettes can cause lung cancer, but few are aware of their close link with heart disease, heart attacks and hypertension. A list of high risk factors predisposing people to cardiovascular disease, based on data drawn from research studies, confirms that cigarette smoking is among the most important of them. Hundreds of clinical trials and aetiological studies have confirmed that there is little doubt about the predictive power of these factors. Estimates based on the Framingham Heart Study and national statistics show us that two out of every three deaths from heart attacks and diseased coronary arteries happen to people exposed to them.

As specialist Robert I. Levy says in 'Prevalence and Epidemiology of Cardiovascular Disease' in Cecil's *Textbook Of Medicine*, edited by James B. Wyngaarden MD and Lloyd H. Smith (Jnr) MD,

> Cigarette smoking has clearly been shown to be an independent, potent risk factor for coronary, cerebral and peripheral vascular disease. Sudden cardiac death, heart attack, angina, claudication, and stroke incidence and prevalence can be related to the number of cigarettes one smokes. The heavier the cigarette smoking history, the higher the risk.

As explained in Chapter 3, peripheral vascular disease has a close association with the development of high blood pressure.

Dr Levy continues:

> Both nicotine and carbon monoxide inhaled with cigarette smoking have been incriminated as causative factors, but definite understanding of cause and effect still eludes us … Furthermore, in contrast to the apparently accumulative relationship of cigarette smoking to lung cancer, a series of prospective and retrospective studies now indicates that if one stops smoking cigarettes, *over 90 per cent of the increased cardiovascular risk disappears within eighteen months* [my italics].

This very encouraging fact should make the effort of quitting smoking worthwhile, as should the recently released information that the effect of smoking upon the coronary arteries (i.e. sending them into spasm) can be triggered for up to eight hours after smoking a single cigarette.

One of the means by which cigarette smoking increases blood pressure is by accelerating the development of atherosclerotic arterial disease. The increased risk of this is plainly shown in the increased incidence of heart attacks, strokes and intermittent claudication seen in smokers – with peripheral vascular disease being the main risk to women. By the age of 45, male smokers run a 70 per cent increased risk of serious disease and death.

Up to the time of the menopause, women receive a certain amount of protection against heart disease and coronary thrombosis from their sex hormones. As their oestrogen levels start to decline (this begins well before menopausal symptoms start) they lose this protection, and over the past 15 years heart attacks have increased by 10 per cent in women as opposed to 3 per cent in men.

Significantly, the rate of smokers among teenage girls has increased and women smokers smoke more heavily than was once the case. As well as favouring blocked, fatty arteries and hypertension, smoking brings on the menopause at an earlier age, thereby hastening the removal of protective oestrogen.

A further effect is an increase in free radical activity in the bodily tissues. Free radicals are electrically charged fragments of molecules produced during normal cellular biochemical processes but capable, when produced in excess, of causing severe tissue damage. Stress (see Chapter 8), atmospheric pollution and other toxic substances also increase free radical manufacture. Among their adverse effects, these molecular fragments increase the risk of degenerative disease such as arthritis and cancer, speed up the ageing process and impair the strength of the immune defence system.

Ironically, vitamin C is a potent fighter of free radical activity, and it is this very vitamin that smoking destroys. In fact, you lose about 25 mg vitamin C for every cigarette you consume.

In addition to tar, cigarette smoke contains over two thousand chemicals, many of which enter the bloodstream through the respiratory surface of the lungs and have a direct effect on vital body organs, including the brain, heart and blood vessels.

Nicotine

Smokers claim that cigarettes 'calm their nerves'. Some studies show that nicotine has a relaxing effect upon body and limb muscles, but its effect upon the central nervous system is excitatory. It enhances the activity of certain enzymes in the liver, where it is largely metabolized, in this way increasing its own rate of breakdown. This accounts, in part, for the development of tolerance to its effects, resulting in the need for an increased number of cigarettes daily.

Nicotine also stimulates the adrenal glands, enhancing their output of the stress hormone adrenaline. This increases sympathetic nervous activity, including the constriction of peripheral blood vessels leading to decreased body temperature and increased blood pressure.

Carbon Monoxide

Present in some commercial gases and produced by the combustion of petrol, this substance is potentially lethal. Suicide resulting from breathing car exhaust fumes results from carbon monoxide poisoning. It affects the haemoglobin (coloured pigment) present in red blood cells, which is responsible for transporting oxygen around the body from the lungs to the tissues and organs.

Under normal conditions, the oxygen we breathe in attaches itself to red cell haemoglobin, forming a compound called oxyhaemoglobin. The bonds between the oxygen and the pigment are loose, and oxygen is readily released in the tissues when necessary.

Carbon monoxide interferes with this process by attaching itself to haemoglobin in place of the oxygen, forming a tightly bonded compound called methoxyhaemoglobin. Death results largely from oxygen starvation.

Cigarettes and Your Brain

While no specific link has yet been proved between cigarette smoking and brain damage similar to that involving alcohol, there is no doubt that the general effects of inhaled cigarette smoke on brain cells are adverse. The brain's oxygen requirement is both high and constant, and clogged cerebral (brain) arteries eventually carry a lower supply of oxygenated blood to the various areas of the brain as atherosclerotic disease progresses. They also become especially prone to damage and clot formation, leading to cerebral haemorrhage and stroke.

Psychologically, many smokers find difficulty in abandoning their habit because cigarettes 'give them something to do with their hands'. Unlikely as this may seem to non-smokers, who unconsciously rely on other body language strategies to give themselves confidence, this can present a major problem to many. Relaxation methods (*see Chapter 8*) are the best solution.

CIGARETTE SMOKING – HOW TO STOP

Chewing gum and skin patches containing nicotine have been available for some years in the UK, Europe and the United States. They can help you give up the habit of smoking, while dampening the withdrawal symptoms from addictive nicotine. Some reports of this therapy show promising results, and the side-effects, which include hiccups, mouth and tongue irritation and heartburn, are generally mild.

A variety of aversion techniques exists. These are based on behaviour modification ideas, stemming from behavioural psychology, and link the act of smoking with an unpleasant experience. Electric aversion therapy, with which many practitioners claim to have a high success rate, applies non-dangerous, although unpleasant, electric shocks to the patient during treatment sessions while he smokes. The idea is that the patient soon links smoking with an unacceptable physical experience, and rapidly grows to dislike it. The technique is easy to carry out, generally inexpensive – at least so far as equipment is concerned – and readily controlled by the therapist.

Rapid smoking therapy involves the patient smoking his or her favourite brand of cigarettes very quickly, at around one puff every six seconds, until he or she can no longer continue. The treatment room is usually decorated with cigarette advertisements, and contains several ashtrays overflowing with offensively smelling cigarette ash and butts. Sometimes electric shocks are administered as well, although many therapists feel that this is unnecessary.

Many studies have shown rapid smoking therapy to have a high success rate, but it can be dangerous to health. It leads to a high blood level of both nicotine and carboxyhaemoglobin (see Carbon monoxide, p 119), which many experts feel make it unsuitable for smokers other than the young and healthy. It is particularly risky for people with clogged coronary arteries and anyone over 35, who may have an existing but undiagnosed heart condition.

Hypnotherapy is also useful. Some hypnotherapists use an aversion technique while the patient is in a state of trance, suggesting to the subconscious mind that cigarettes will henceforth taste of something particularly unpleasant. Others rely more upon ego boosting, i.e. confidence building, getting the message through to the patient's subconscious mind that he or she will from then on feel relaxed rather than tense in stressful situations, when socializing etc., and that the need to smoke will rapidly diminish. Some therapists succeed with a single consultation and hypnotherapy session only.

Others use the 'Q-day' technique. This consists of four hypnotherapy/ counselling sessions, usually at seven-day intervals, during which cigarette consumption is reduced by an amount mutually agreed between therapist and patient until Q-day, that is quitting day, is reached, by the final session.

You may need some kind of therapeutic aid to quit smoking. On the other hand, you may decide to 'go it alone'. Rather than trying to reinforce your willpower which can lead to increased tension, an increased need for cigarettes and failure, master a relaxation technique before you stop, and damp down sympathetic nervous activity under stressful conditions, particularly when withdrawal symptoms are getting to you, by putting the technique into practice. It is also helpful to set aside the money you normally waste on cigarettes every week, and use it to offset outstanding bills which anyway increase your tension or, if possible, save it up for a special treat for you, your partner or family.

ALCOHOL AND HIGH BLOOD PRESSURE

A research paper published in the German cardiology journal *Heiz* in 1996 by heart specialist Professor H. Rupp *et al.* discussed the deleterious effects of heavy drinking on blood pressure via a number of heart and blood-vessel related mechanisms. In February 1999, the American journal *Alcoholism: Clinical & Experimental Research* discussed heavy alcohol consumption as a major risk factor in developing hypertension. And the WHO International Society of Hypertension: Guidelines for Managing Hypertension 1999 (updated February 2001) acknowledged the beneficial effects of 2–3 alcoholic drinks a day (reduces risk of coronary heart disease by 30–40 per cent) but pointed out that heavy – especially binge – drinking greatly increases the risks of heart disease, hypertension and stroke.

ALCOHOL AND YOUR BODY

Besides generating high blood pressure, alcohol abuse leads to other cardiovascular problems. These include heart palpitations, abnormal heart rhythms and sudden death, and chronic damage to the muscle of the heart leading to an increasing degree of heart failure.

Alcohol abuse also affects other bodily systems. It causes fatty infiltration of the liver, hepatitis, cirrhosis and eventual liver failure, and the formation of liver tumours (hepatoma). It affects the stomach and intestinal system by causing irritation to the stomach lining (gastritis), diarrhoea, disease of the pancreas, poor food absorption and overweight; and it increases the risk of cancer of the food pipe (oesophagus). Heavy drinkers also run an increased risk of lung disease, especially chemical pneumonia, due to inhalation of vomit when in an alcoholic stupor. Alcohol abuse in women leads to sexual problems, irregular periods, and shrinkage of breasts and the external genitals; in men, it can cause loss of sex drive, reduced potency, a reduced or absent sperm count and infertility, and shrinkage of the penis and testes.

ALCOHOL AND YOUR BRAIN

Alcohol abuse can inflict persistent brain damage. Various parts of the brain can degenerate, leading to dementia, and it increases the risk of brain blood vessel disease, including bleeding episodes (subarachnoid haemorrhage), strokes – especially in young people – and the formation of blood clots in the brain following head injury.

Other effects on the nervous system include weakness, paralysis and tingling/pins and needles in the hands and feet. Withdrawal symptoms include fits, hallucinations and trembling of the hands.

Psychiatric illness is common in alcohol abusers. Anxiety neurosis and severe depression are common, as are loss of memory (amnesia) and sleeping problems. Depression, suicidal tendencies, anxiety and insomnia bring in their wake problems at work and home. Rows, physical and verbal violence, absenteeism, inefficiency, loss of interest in everyday affairs and relationships, and divorce also commonly result.

WHAT CONSTITUTES ABUSE?

A unit of alcohol is defined in standard units, where one unit is equivalent to half a pint of beer, a four-ounce glass of table wine, a glass of sherry, or a single whisky, gin or other form of spirits. Social drinkers are usually defined as people who drink no more than two to three units of alcohol daily, don't become intoxicated, and aren't likely to harm themselves or their family. Moderate drinkers regularly consume more than five units of alcohol a day, although apparently without immediate harm. The amount of alcohol we, as individuals, can take differs widely, with respect to its effects upon us and our lives, and problem drinkers are defined as people who experience physical, psychological, social, family, occupational, financial or legal problems directly attributable to drinking, regardless of the amount.

Dependent drinkers consume roughly the same quantity of alcohol each day. Drinking is the most important factor in their lives, and many quit the habit only to resume it after a period of abstinence. They tend to have an increased tolerance to alcohol in the early stages of dependence, and reduced tolerance later on. They experience withdrawal symptoms when deprived of alcohol, which they relieve by drinking more.

Signs of dependence to watch out for include a growing preoccupation with alcohol, combined with defensiveness about consumption, early morning drinking, and the feeling of absolute necessity to get a drink. Character changes include increasing aggressiveness, denial and anger if tackled on the subject, and increasing absenteeism from work.

Alcohol consumption is increasing in children and adolescents – a finding of many studies including one conducted from 1997–2000 by researchers at the Universities of Wales (Swansea) and Leeds, UK. A major trigger seems to be the easy availability of alcopops and other sorts of alcohol. The majority (61.1 per cent) of the 4,516 11–16-year-olds drank alcohol *regularly* (i.e. had drunk alcohol weekly for the past three months). This is consistent with the results of another recent UK study (Balding, 1997) that 50 per cent of 12–13-year-old British adolescents are regular drinkers; and with a Welsh study which found that 65 per cent of 15–16-year-old boys and 54 per cent of girls drink alcohol on a regular (weekly) basis.

WHO IS AT RISK?

All but teetotallers run some risk of becoming alcohol abusers, and the safest advice to follow is to avoid alcohol when you are depressed, anxious, stressed or tired. However much tension and fatigue may increase your desire to 'tipple', your body and brain can become used to the soothing effects of a glass of sherry, wine or beer far sooner than you may realize.

As a nation the British are drinking more than they were a decade ago, and over that period women in particular have increased their alcohol consumption.

HOW TO STOP EXCESSIVE DRINKING

An alcohol abuser in the family is a sick person and requires urgent help, but the problems he or she can cause to other family members would be hard to exaggerate. The organization, Alateen, helps young people whose parents or close relatives are alcohol dependent, while Al-Anon helps the families of alcoholics. For help and information about local branches, contact Alcoholics Anonymous, which you will find listed in local telephone directories and the Yellow Pages (*see also below*).

Some hospitals have special units and a number of private clinics offer medical treatment and counselling. Your GP should be able to give you the information you require about local facilities. The national drink watchers network, with branches throughout the country, offers advice and help on monitoring individual drinking patterns. The best-known organization, Alcoholics Anonymous, can be contacted at General Service

Office, P.O. Box 1, Stonebow House, Stonebow, York YO1 2NJ. Tel. (01904) 644026/7/8/9. Alcohol Concern, based at 305 Gray's Inn Road, London WC1X 8QF, tel. (0207) 833 3471, provides information about help with drinking problems available nationally and locally. In the USA, Alcoholics Anonymous are based at 468 Park Avenue South, New York, NY 10016; tel. (212) 686 1100. Elsewhere, check the Yellow Pages.

Chapter ten

Alternative Therapies

Complementary medicine has become increasingly widely used over the past 20 years; it is now estimated that one in three Britons has used some form of it. According to a survey published in the *British Medical Journal*, the six most popular therapies are acupuncture, herbal medicine, homoeopathy, hypnotherapy, chiropractic and osteopathy, and the first four have been used successfully to treat high blood pressure and related problems (obesity, compulsive eating, anxiety and panic disorders, angina and addictive cravings).

Medical herbalism needs special mention. Not only has it been the main source of medical treatment for many millions of people both in Europe and other parts of the world since time immemorial, it has also provided the foundation upon which modern pharmaceutical knowledge has developed into a vital and highly sophisticated science.

However, much still remains to be understood about complementary therapies and their underlying philosophy. Many people remain sceptical about the value of piercing the skin of the ear lobe with an acupuncture needle, for example, in order to relieve food cravings and withdrawal symptoms from cigarette smoking. Homoeopathy is still ridiculed by those who, while not denying that like may well cure like, doubt that the potency of homoeopathic remedies is inversely proportional to the amount of active substance they contain. And reflexology – pressure applied to the soles of the feet at certain predetermined points – strikes many newcomers to alternative medicine as an odd way to relieve backache, peptic ulcer pain or eczema.

The main thing to remember about alternative therapies is that they are based on an alternative view of how the body functions. Conventional medicine sees disease in terms of direct cause and effect, and treats cystitis, for example, with antibiotics to kill bacteria, and a head cold with aspirin to relieve the fever and inflammation. Alternative practitioners, by contrast, take a broader, i.e. holistic, view and attribute illness to a disturbance in the overall harmony that exists in a healthy person, between body, mind and spirit.

Alternative therapies aim to discover the reason for the causative imbalance and to redress it wherever possible. They recognize the existence of the life force, which they equate with the principle differentiating living from non-living matter, and state that its potency depends upon the harmony and the smooth co-operation of all those parts, physical and ethereal, of which we are composed. Although conventional medicine can offer specific treatments – in particular, drugs – for the vast majority of ailments, the alternatives, based upon a broader philosophy, use a relatively small number of corrective techniques.

The concept of the life force, and the rationale of manoeuvres to restore its strength, have been the focus of most of the controversy separating orthodox and complementary medicine. Yet with the advent of increasing evidence in support of the reality of the life force, and the success achieved by complementary therapists in cases where conventional medicine has failed, the dichotomy is being steadily bridged. Doctors who add acupuncture to the treatments they offer their patients may not think of this discipline in terms of freeing clogged channels (meridians) along which the life force flows, but the medical profession as a whole is paying increasing attention to objective scientific evidence supporting the interdependence of mind and body, and the possible adverse effects of one upon the other.

Alternative practitioners attribute great importance to the effects of the emotions on the human organism, and counselling plays a major role in many of their therapies. Traditionally, medical doctors set less store on talking and listening than upon prescribing medicines and tablets. Recent research has shown, however, that the immune defence system, our main means of protection against invading bacteria and viruses, malignant cell change and premature ageing, is weakened by stress, anxiety and depression – and that we become more susceptible to both infectious illness and cancer when persistently tense and unhappy.

Circumstantial proof of this kind has already gone a long way towards emphasizing the vital interplay between body, mind and spirit. As research reveals further evidence of this nature, orthodox doctors will inevitably grow closer to an understanding and an acceptance of the alternative view. And, as in all balanced systems, there are advantages to both sides. Many complementary practitioners are coming to feel the need to base the therapies they practise upon a more scientific and disciplined basis. This does not mean that reflexology, for instance, lacks veracity because its effectiveness cannot be demonstrated under laboratory conditions, but it recognizes the value of scientific and clinical trials wherever these are applicable, and the need to establish properly organized training courses for future therapists.

Most of the alternative therapies can prove useful in cases of hypertension, either in helping to reduce it in a direct sense, or in combating adverse factors such as stress, high blood-fat levels, alcohol and tobacco withdrawal symptoms, and high blood weight. We have already looked at relaxation methods; in this final chapter, we will see what medical herbalism, homoeopathy, traditional Chinese medicine, hypnotherapy and naturopathy have to offer.

MEDICAL HERBALISM

Herbal medicine – or, to give it the name many practitioners favour, medical herbalism – is at first difficult to equate with the concept of complementary or alternative medicine. So naturally and imperceptibly has this age-old form of medical practice given rise to current pharmaceutical science and industry that the temptation arises to regard it simply as the worthy but anachronistic precursor of modern drug therapy.

This view is, in fact, grossly unjust to the art and science of medical herbalism which flourishes, and will continue to flourish, as a major and significant form of complementary medicine in its own right. That its foundations are rooted in the earliest attempts to combat disease needs no emphasis here. Certainly, modern pharmacy owes an incalculable debt to the wisdom and expertise of herbal practitioners throughout history; but the fact that medical herbalism has continued to offer enormous benefits to the sick in every race is indisputable.

At a scientific level, herbal preparations can be seen as a source of the essential vitamins, minerals and trace elements needed to promote health and combat disease. At a more comprehensive level, the medicinal substances used by practitioners, culled as they are from whole, living plants, contain within them a complete range of active ingredients co-existing in a harmonious and natural state. According to medical herbalists, it is the state of balance inherent in herbal remedies, as much as the constituents themselves, that is responsible for their curative properties.

Medical herbalists take stock of a patient's presenting symptoms, but attach more importance to his/her overall state of integrated balance and harmony. Their aim is to identify underlying imbalances in the various bodily and psychological systems to reach a diagnosis, and to treat the whole person by restoring him/her to a state of equilibrium. This explains why different remedies may be employed to treat the same condition in different patients; for, like other complementary therapists, medical herbalists aim at treating the complete person as an individual being.

Practitioners of herbal medicine oppose the extraction of a single, active element from a medicinal plant. They view this strategy as highly conducive to the production of adverse side-effects – an opinion borne out by many recipients of orthodox medicine. Digoxin, for example, prescribed for heart failure, can have serious side-effects when used as a drug. Foxglove extract, by contrast, contains within it a range of natural ingredients which combat heart failure yet, when prescribed judiciously by a competent herbalist, are less inclined to cause adverse reactions.

Herbal remedies for self-administration abound, and are easily accessible, yet they should be taken in strict accordance with the instructions provided. They are no more a 'panacea for all ills' than are vitamins, minerals and other natural supplements, and since they are sufficiently potent to relieve, and often cure, diseases, it follows that their misuse can result in serious consequences.

Most medical herbalists emphasize the importance of consulting a qualified practitioner about all but the most trivial ailments. Treatment for high blood pressure would be aimed in the first instance at the underlying problem of small blood vessel constriction and disease, accompanied by advice about lifestyle changes, stress reduction, exercise and diet.

Likely remedies would be those with vasodilatory effect, i.e. those capable of relaxing the narrowed walls of the peripheral blood vessels. Important examples include limeflowers, hawthorn and garlic, because of their ability to improve the circulation and tissue oxygenation. These may be prescribed in combination with diuretic herbs, such as parsley, celery, dandelion leaves, wild carrot and asparagus; and natural relaxants, such as rosemary, lavender, lemon balm, chamomile and catmint. Substantial falls in blood pressure are often obtained by these measures.

Ancient Indian medical philosophy has enjoyed increasing popularity recently. Ayurvedic herbal remedies – Rasayanas – aim to balance the body and mind and effect rejuvenation in a curative sense to the nerves and blood vessels. Among the herbal extracts used in this way are garlic, gotu kola, skullcap and valerian, cinnamon and burdock and, for the preparation of herbal tablets, hawthorn, kelp and cardamom.

Most manufacturers spell out the fact that their preparations have been used for many hundreds of years, but (in the main) they have not been subjected to scientific trials. For this reason, I would urge caution in their use, and consultation with an experienced Ayurvedic practitioner. Suggested benefits include reduced blood pressure, tension and stress, improved sleep, calming of the nerves, and strengthening and calming of the heart muscle.

HOMOEOPATHIC MEDICINE

Homoeopathy as a system of medicine originated in the research of Dr Samuel Hahnemann, an 18th-century German physician and chemist. Two prime factors motivated his search for an alternative method of treating patients. The first was his dissatisfaction with orthodox medicine's tendency to treat symptoms rather than patients as individuals. The second was his dislike of the barbarous treatment methods then in fashion. Bleeding, purging and powerful emetics (to provoke vomiting), stimulants and sedatives were all commonly employed, together with surgery which as yet knew the benefits of neither anaesthesia nor hygiene.

Like naturopathic practitioners, Hahnemann believed in the body's ability to heal itself, and regarded symptoms as evidence of attempts to put that healing ability into practice. In his famous work, *The Organon Of Rational Healing* (1810), he described the vital force which he held responsible for the body's natural healing processes. Again in common with naturopathic philosophy, he was convinced that disease resulted from inner disharmony, and believed that treatment should aim at restoring balance between the physical, mental and spiritual aspects of human nature.

Biochemistry was one of Hahnemann's particular interests. Using a wide range of natural remedies derived from animal, plant and mineral origins, and himself as guinea pig, he rediscovered a principle of medicine whose validity had been recognized since the time of Hippocrates. This principle states that 'like cures like'. He started by experimenting with currently used drugs, the difference being that in taking them himself he was using them on a healthy rather than on a sick person.

He discovered that the substances he took produced the symptoms he would have expected had he been suffering from the illness they were normally employed to cure. Quinine, used for malaria, was a case in point. He took sizeable doses for two days, and found that his extremities grew cold; that he became sleepy and exhausted; that his pulse raced, and that he experienced palpitations. He felt extremely anxious, trembled all over, his head throbbed, his face grew flushed and he felt extremely thirsty. Having had malaria earlier in life, he was able to confirm the effects of the quinine to resemble those of the illness very closely.

He concluded from this that quinine overpowered malarial fever by creating a fever of its own, and that the symptoms of the illness were not evidence of the disease itself but of the body's resistance to it. Using both himself and healthy volunteer subjects to discover whether this principle would be borne out in other instances, he was eventually able to confirm that a drug which produced certain symptoms in healthy people was the drug of choice to treat those symptoms when patients became ill.

Just as vaccination with, for example, a tiny quantity of tetanus toxoid causes the immune defence system to produce antibodies against further encounters with the tetanus bacteria, so homoeopathic remedies stimulate the body's inherent healing capacity. Hahnemann soon discovered, too, that the smaller the dose, the greater the effect. Various theories have been put forward to account for this apparent anomaly; and the explanation now seems to lie in the method used in preparing the remedies.

'Mother tinctures' – alcoholic extracts of the plant, mineral or other substance used – are made, and repeatedly diluted (i.e. triturated) a hundredfold. The first dilution is termed 1C; the second, 2C, is a hundredth dilution of the first, i.e. the original tincture diluted 10,000 times. The preparation is then 'succussed' i.e. shaken vigorously by hand or machine many times over. It is this process that is believed to 'potentize' the remedy being prepared, probably by increasing the molecular energy of the active substances it contains. What the patient finally receives is the active substance in a very low concentration but in a state of high energy.

In addition to taking a formal case history, homoeopathic practitioners ask their patients many questions that can, on face value, seem irrelevant. They might want to know whether the symptoms are more troublesome in cold weather or when milk is taken, or whether the individual likes or fears the dark, loud noises or thunderstorms. Importance is also attached to personality, physical appearance, hair colour, skin colour etc. Homoeopaths need this information in order to match the remedies they use as closely as possible to the person they are treating. This is why the same symptoms, e.g. sneezing, fever, sore throat, in three very different patients may be treated with different remedies, picked in each case to conform to the individual as a whole person. Similarly, the same remedy may be selected to treat widely differing symptoms in patients of similar types.

There is plenty of evidence that scientifically-conducted studies of homoeopathic treatment are being carried out, yet, in common with other branches of complementary medicine, some orthodox doctors still reiterate the same, lame old complaint: 'There are no properly-conducted studies so we can't pass a professional opinion on it!' It's time we all woke up and sniffed the coffee (a commonly used homoeopathic remedy, by the way – but not for hypertension).

Here are some of the most frequently-mentioned remedies for treating people with high blood pressure:

Sanguinaria: might be selected by a homoeopathic doctor for a patient complaining of blood rushing to the head, with flushed red cheeks and pulsing in the neck. Also headaches and migraines (usually on the right, aggravated by light and noise), right-sided neck and shoulder problems, allergies, heartburn and other digestive problems. Craving for spicy foods and tendency to feel worse after eating sweets.

Nux vomica: typical recipient may be sensitive and emotional, strongly desiring sweets, coffee and other stimulants, strong foods, alcohol or drugs, which aggravate BP problems; sensitive to light, noise, odours and interference, and complaining of tightness in the chest, piles and constipation.

Argentum nitricum: if blood pressure rises with anxiety and nervousness; anticipation of a frightening experience (stage fright) triggers dizziness, headaches, diarrhoea and a pounding pulse. Recipients typically impulsive and warm-blooded, imaginative and claustrophobic, often strongly craving salt and sweet things.

Belladonna: indicated for symptoms that come on suddenly, with great intensity and heat. Person's face is flushed, with large pupils, and throbbings experienced in various parts of the body. Vertigo and pounding headaches, worsened by jarring movements and bright lights.

Like herbal medicines, homoeopathic remedies for serious conditions such as high blood pressure are better prescribed by a qualified practitioner than used for self-treatment.

TRADITIONAL CHINESE MEDICINE

This comprehensive, highly detailed system of medical practice has little in common with Western medicine apart from the will, and the ability, to heal. Acupuncture is more familiar to most of us than, say, Chinese herbalism and Qi Dong (a form of meditation for energy balance), and a brief account of its development and theory are illustrative of TCM as a whole.

The origins of acupuncture are uncertain, but evidence exists that it was practised in China as long ago as the third millennium BC. Huan Ti, who became Emperor of China and was known as the Father of Acupuncture, worked together with his personal physician Ch'i Po to establish the principles of anatomy, health and disease upon which this medical art is based. Huan Ti described his findings in *Nei Ching* (the Yellow Emperor's Classic of Internal Medicine), a book that remained the definitive authority on the subject for many centuries.

Like other forms of holistic medicine, acupuncture sees disease as the result of disharmony, in particular of blockage of the life force, ch'i, which is considered to pass along invisible lines known as meridians running throughout the body. Two great life elements called yin and yang, complementary opposites, remain in a state of balance when a person is healthy, permitting ch'i to flow freely along the meridian lines. But when yin and yang become unbalanced, through inherent weakness, stress, the effects of toxins and other adverse factors, ch'i's flow is impeded, giving rise to the symptoms of illness.

Yin and yang are elements in all traditional Eastern philosophies. They are polar opposites, present in all things, and can be discerned throughout nature at every juncture. Examples include the male and female principles, coldness and heat, wetness and dryness, hardness and softness, dominance and receptivity, activity and passivity, positive and negative, light and darkness, day and night.

Like other comparable systems, yin and yang exist in a state of mutual but dynamic equilibrium, which exists as a coherent and live 'whole', elements of each principle fluctuating while the complete system remains in a state of balance. When adverse factors such as those mentioned above upset the state of equilibrium, allowing either yin or yang to hold sway over the other, the effects are felt at the level of the life force, and the living organism suffers accordingly.

The object of an acupuncturist is to identify the underlying problem and to treat it by removing the obstruction to ch'i's free flow, thereby restoring harmony and health. He or she takes a detailed case history, examines the patient, considers the relevant organs in terms of their yin and yang characteristics, determines the meridian lines involved, and completes the diagnosis by taking the pulses at each wrist – a far more complex and detailed enterprise than pulse examination in conventional medicine.

Treatment consists of stimulating certain high energy points (i.e. acupuncture points) along the meridian lines by means of needles, heat (moxibustion), and/or modern innovations such as electromagnetic energy, polarized light, low power lasers and tuning forks vibrating at a certain required resonance. Its effect is to unblock the clogged meridian(s) and restore yin and yang to harmonious and integrated balance.

Acupuncture was first heard of in Europe in the 17th century, when missionaries from China told of its practice on their return to the West. A few Chinese specialists practised it in the UK in the early part of the 20th century, but it did not become known to the general public until the late 1950s. With the great growth of interest in alternative medicine in the 1960s and 1970s, acupuncture flourished and became widely practised.

Its frequent successes naturally caused much controversy. Initially, most orthodox doctors were highly sceptical, and attributed cures to that well-known panacea for many ills, the placebo effect. Later, research was carried out on volunteers under scientifically controlled conditions, and the existence of both meridian lines and acupuncture points was supported by considerable evidence.

Acupuncture is now practised in Britain by both medically qualified doctors and by lay therapists. Not all practitioners necessarily subscribe – or even understand – the basic Chinese philosophy involving ch'i, yin and yang; but results continue to justify the growing popularity of this form of alternative medicine.

It can help in cases of hypertension by reducing the blood pressure reading, although the beneficial effects often require 'top up' treatment sessions if they are to be maintained. It can help withdrawal symptoms from both tobacco and alcohol, and has permitted many longtime smokers to give up the habit. Beyond doubt, acupuncture has a harmonizing and energizing effect on mind and body, and can help food cravings in overweight people as well as anxiety and tension.

Numerous studies of acupuncture's efficacy in patients with blood pressure have been carried out over the past 10 years. One study reported in the *Journal of Traditional Chinese Medicine* in 1992 (1) involved 30 patients with Grades II and III hypertension, and compared the auricular (i.e. ear) stimulation of the Heart acupuncture point with that of the Stomach (to establish a 'control'). While the latter had no blood pressure-lowering effect, stimulation of the Heart point markedly reduced BP and improved cardiac function in every case immediately following treatment, and effectively reduced BP in 63.3 per cent of patients long term

Similarly, a German study in 1990 treated 98 hypertensive patients with auricular electroacupuncture, relieving 66 per cent of those with Grade I and 57 per cent of those with Grade II, allowing the former to stop taking their medication and the latter to reduce their doses. Another study from the Hospital of Oriental Medicine, Seoul, Korea, examined the effects of acupuncture on 22 stroke patients with mild hypertension who were not taking blood pressure medication. Blood pressure monitored over 24 hours with an ambulatory BP device before and after treatment found that auricular acupuncture significantly reduced systolic and diastolic BPs equally in men and women and without significantly changing the heart rate.

HYPNOTHERAPY

Research trials of the efficacy of hypnotherapy in treating hypertension are not easy to find but, as a trained hypnotherapist, I can say that the potential for success is enormous. Compatibility between subject and therapist is, of course, essential – they must feel comfortable working together and, having had any doubts or fears dispelled before the start of the first session, the subject must want the treatment to work. This may sound obvious, particularly given the price some people are willing pay for treatment, but hidden resistance to suggestions to the subconscious mind is one of the commonest causes of failure.

Nevertheless, hypnotherapy has an overall success rate of around 80 per cent (meaning therapists succeed in inducing trance in around eight out of ten subjects, and that the subject subsequently benefits, for a time at least, from some of the sought-after effects). In a case of hypertension, a therapist would be likely to include suggestions that the subject remain calm in future when in a stressful situation; and he/she might also employ guided imagery and constructive visualization similar to that used to assist cancer patients gain the upper hand of their illness.

When calm, relaxed and in a medium-light trance, the therapist would take the person on an imaginary journey to a pleasant, tranquil setting such as a sunny field or woodland waterfall and then get them to 'lie down', feel the sun on their face and visualize their high blood pressure and any attendant symptoms gradually subsiding. Graphic images, such as of constricted blood vessels opening up and relaxing, would be used to help the subject achieve this, and future success would very likely depend, at least in part, on regular repetitions of this exercise at home.

NATUROPATHY

Naturopathic medicine is a complete and distinct form of medicine which concentrates upon the body's inherent capacity for self-healing and self-repair. Its aim is to create suitable conditions for this to take place. The name 'naturopathy' has been used since the turn of the century, but the philosophy underlying the system and many of its methods date back to at least 400 BC and were practised by Hippocrates.

There are three basic tenets of naturopathy:

(1) Only nature heals. It does so by the life force re-establishing harmony and balance, provided we make this possible.

(2) Disease results from the body's attempt to remove impediments to the normal working of its tissues and organs. These impediments are classified into three types: chemical, mechanical and psychological. Chemical problems refer to aspects of the body's biochemistry, i.e. poor nutrition, inefficient excretion of waste matter through the bowels, kidneys, lungs, skin etc.

Mechanical problems responsible for ill-health include stiff joints, weak or tense muscles, bad posture and misalignment of the spinal vertebrae, leading to musculoskeletal and nervous system ailments.

The implication of this latter point is wide. Misaligned vertebrae can affect the spinal cord, the messages it carries between the brain and the rest of the body, and the parasympathetic and sympathetic ganglia or nerve centres controlling the autonomic nervous system and thereby factors such as the contraction and expansion of blood vessels, the blood pressure etc.

Psychological problems include all the possible adverse effects of stress, anxiety, depression from whatever cause, upon the body and its organs.

(3) The third tenet of naturopathy has already been explained in the discussion about the principal differences between the orthodox and alternative approaches to health and disease. That is, that disease arises from disharmony between body, mind and spirit, and affects the whole body regardless of the fact that overt symptoms may suggest that simply one organ is diseased.

The individuality of each person is regarded as highly important, and the nature of that individuality is held to be partly responsible for his or her health. Each of us possesses certain strengths and weaknesses, and reacts differently under strain. This is why naturopathic practitioners take carefully detailed case histories, and attach considerable importance to inherited defects, the possibility of pre-birth trauma, and the individual's environment.

During a consultation, discussion is followed by a physical examination and relevant biochemical investigations of, for example, urine, blood, sputum (phlegm), secretions etc. Once a diagnosis is reached in the light of all the information gained, the naturopath sets out to decide how best the patient can be helped to help him- or herself.

In dealing with a case of high blood pressure, special importance would be attached to past medical history, health/causes of death of parents and/or close relatives, the state of the heart and circulatory system, the function of the autonomic nervous system, and present/recent stresses, strains, emotional problems and social habits.

Treatment would focus upon diet and weight control along the lines discussed in Chapter 5; advice would be given regarding smoking and alcohol consumption with, perhaps, referral to an acupuncturist or hypnotherapist if extra help were required. Many naturopaths favour fasting as a means of treatment, and this may be suggested, and carried out, with the patient's co-operation, under the therapist's guidance.

Relaxation techniques and exercise regimens would be recommended, perhaps in combination with therapeutic massage. Advice would be given about poor posture, and how it could be rectified. Many naturopathic practitioners practise other forms of alternative medicine in addition to their own. Those skilled in osteopathy might treat spinal misalignment personally, while others would refer their patient to another therapist.

While drugs are regarded essentially as undesirable toxins, no patient would be told by an experienced naturopath to cease taking prescribed medication forthwith. Herbal remedies and dietary supplements compatible with current treatment may well be recommended, but the aim of naturopathic practitioners is to ease the body into a state of health so that, in so far as it is possible, drugs either become unnecessary or can be utilized in smaller doses.

Useful Addresses

The British Naturopathic and Osteopathic Association, Goswell House, 2 Goswell Road, Street, Somerset BA16 0JG; tel. (01458) 840072

Society of Homoeopaths, 2 Artizan Road, Northampton NN1 4HU; tel. (01604) 621400

British Acupuncture Association and Register, 34 Alderney Street, London SW1V 4EU; tel. (0207) 834 1012

The British Acupuncture Council, Park House, 206–208 Latimer Road, London W10 6RE; tel. (0208) 964 0222

National Council of Psychotherapists and Hypnotherapists, 1 Clovelly Road, Ealing, London W5

Professional associations outside the UK

Outside the UK, you should be able to obtain addresses from the Yellow Pages, but here are some suggestions for the USA and Australia:

American Association of Naturopathic Physicians, 900 Madison Street, Seattle, WA 98104 (206 328-7971)

Traditional Acupuncture Foundation, American City Building, Columbia,
   MD 21044
International Foundation for Homoeopathy, 2366 Eastlake East, No. 301,
   Seattle, WA 98102 (206 324-8230)
Australian Natural Therapeutic Association, 31 Victoria Street, Fitzroy,
   Melbourne
Australian Traditional Medicine Society, Rozelle, Victoria
Australian Homoeopathic Association, c/o 16a Edward Street, Gordon,
   NSW 2027
National Herbalists Association of Australia, 27 Leith Street, Cooparoo,
   Queensland 4151

Index

seven-day eating plan 70–84
sex differences 33, 49–50, 118, 123
side-effects 4, 5–11, 13, 14
skullcap 131
sleep 101
Slow-Trasicor 6
Slozem 8
smoking 16, 49–50, 116–22
snacks 71
sport 45
    see also exercise
statins 31
stepped care treatment 51–3
streptokinase 46
steroids 29
Stobhill General Hospital 16
stress 32, 33, 34, 42, 86, 93–5, 100, 107
stroke 4, 37, 39–40
sugar, in diet 69, 86
supplements, see dietary supplements
Swales, Prof John 15
swimming 98, 103
sympathetic nervous system 32, 109–10

tablets, taking, problems 13–14
taurine 89
Tenormin 6
Tensipine-MR 8
Thiaver 10
thiazides 5, 31, 49
thrombosis (blood clots) 42, 43, 99
thyrotoxicosis 28
Tildiem 8
timolol 31
toxaemia of pregnancy 28–9
traditional Chinese medicine 135–8
Trandate 11, 51
transcendental meditation 114
transient ischaemic attacks 40
Trasicor 6

Trasidrex 6
treatment 36–7, 47–56
    see also alternative treatment; drug
        treatment
Triam-Co 6
triamterene 6
trimetaphan 10
Turnbull, Nancy 99
Type A personality 99–100

Univer 7

valerian 131
valsartan 9
vasodilators 7, 15, 52, 55
    herbal 131
vegetables 64, 68, 85
vegetarian diet 67
veins 22
verapamil 7
veratrum 10
Veriloid 10
vitamin B complex 94
vitamin C 93–4, 119
vitamin E 87–8

walking 98, 103
water pills, see diuretics
weight control 34, 60–1
    see also obesity
whole foods 61–84, 85
wild carrot 131
women 33, 46, 49–50, 118, 123

yoga 114

Zemtard XL 8
Zestril 8
zinc 95